CONTENTS

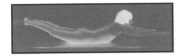

Beginner Level Lessons

Intermediate Level Lessons

Advanced Level 1 Lessons

Advanced Level 2 Lessons

Advanced Level 3 Lessons

ACKNOWLEDGMENTS

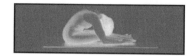

There was once a source of clay with all the necessary ingredients to become something useful to those who availed themselves of it. As qualitative as the clay was, its value was diminished without a potter to construct it into a finished form and to add a touch of dignity and beauty. *Yoga for Real People* is of this origin. I was but the clay. Diane Peck was the potter, and for this, I am most grateful. I would also like to thank Jennie Sabato for allowing me to put her into these positions so I would know they are correct, Moto Photo for their professionalism in photography, and Valerie Cooper for her careful restoration of parts lost.

INTRODUCTION

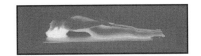

THE PATH TO COMPLETE HEALTH

What is yoga? Is it really lying on a bed of nails, walking on water, or being buried alive? Of course not, except for advanced students, perhaps. There are many types of yogas: Hatha Yoga, Raja Yoga, Karma Yoga, Jnana Yoga, Mantra Yoga, Bhakti Yoga, and Kundalini Yoga.

Hatha Yoga gives us a second chance at life. You can practice yoga at any age. If you want to live longer, be healthier and more at peace, yoga has the answer. How long will it take you to accomplish this? That's up to you. If you only practice once a week, then it may take you a very long time. However, if you are more dedicated and recognize the importance of the three "Ds"—desire, dedication, and discipline— there is no limit to what you can accomplish. Each person is different, and your progress is completely up to you. Yoga is not a miracle practice, but it is common sense. It is a preventive, not a cure.

Hatha Yoga is the combination of postures and breathing working together. The asanas (the postures) give us strength, and the mudras (positions of the hands and fingers) add balance and steadiness to our lives. *Ha* means "Sun." *Tha* means "Moon." Hatha Yoga is truly solar-lunar yoga. The right side of your body is positive—the Sun, heat, masculine. The left side of your body is negative—the Moon, cool, feminine. Yoga brings these together in perfect balance and harmony.

Yoga is six thousand years old. Of its 840,000 postures, 48 are basic, 32 are beneficial, and 10 are essential and should be practiced every day. All postures should be performed slowly. We stretch, we do not strain. We use our body, we do not abuse it.

There are basically three types of postures. Stretching postures, such as the Cat, improve our body's flexibility and elasticity. They are especially beneficial for our tendons and ligaments. Inversion postures, such as the Plow, stimulate our glands and circulation. They refresh our brain and improve our complexion. Finally, sitting postures in combination with pranayama breathing calm our metabolism and nerves and increase our lung capacity, as well as our vitality. We must breathe properly with each posture. Practiced correctly, yoga tends to normalize the functions of our entire body; it regulates our respiration, our circulation, our digestion, our elimination, and our metabolism.

Many forms of exercise are practiced quickly, violently, and make us tired and sore. Sometimes, rough exercise can cause injuries. You may even want to give it up after a while. Yoga is the complete opposite to this kind of practice. It is known as the "gentle" form of exercise. When practiced correctly and regularly, it strengthens the muscles, keeps the spine flexible, loosens stiff or aching joints, calms the mind, and brings balance and harmony to the whole being. Yoga builds energy, while it relaxes you and massages all your organs.

Your success with yoga depends on two things: regular practice and progress. Continue searching for yourself, from beginner's yoga, to intermediate yoga, to advanced yoga. There's always something new for you to learn, and your body is always in need of being moved and stretched gently, just as your mind is always in need of rest and your spirit in need of inspiration.

As with any form of exercise, you should learn to pay attention to your own body because nobody knows your body better than you do. During your yoga practice, and after each posture, pay close attention to how your body reacts to past injuries or physical discomfort. You must learn to listen to your body. Your body communicates with you, and every movement affects your entire body. There are no isolated movements. Every twinge, every feeling of stretch, pull, and pain is a statement. Listen to it! If discomfort or pain arises in your practice, you should stop immediately and analyze what it is that you are feeling: Have you stretched too far, beyond your own level of comfort? Have you moved into a posture too quickly, without paying attention to the feel of your body?

Yoga for Real People is not just another book of postures and breathing techniques. Basically, it is a year of classes with a yoga teacher. This book is intended to act as a guide for dedicated students who are interested in furthering their growth. It presents complete lessons for beginning to advanced levels of practice. I discuss all aspects of health in the hope that it may help you become a more complete person, take your own well-being into your own hands, and be at peace with yourself.

The book is divided into five sections: Beginners Level, Intermediates Level, and Advanced Level I, II, and III. Each lesson, within each section, presents an opening discussion, a series of postures, presented in the order in which they should be performed, and a closing relaxation/meditation period. The book's appendix and index will guide you through the complete list of postures, as well as some of the benefits of each posture.

As a beginner, you will simply "do" one posture at a time, stopping between each one, and learn to become aware of your body and the effects of the postures. At the intermediate level, you'll learn how to "experience" the postures. With Lesson 7, you'll commence practicing continuities, which are groups of postures performed one after another, without pausing, to create an uninterrupted flow of movement. Continuities are practiced in related groups intended to provide a fully balanced practice. You'll eventually begin to learn how to flow with the postures, no longer recognizing the end of one and the beginning of another. As an advanced student, you'll learn to "become" the posture, as you move into one continual flow of movement and being-ness. At this level, you are the posture. As with all the postures in this book, it is important that those in the continuities be practiced *in the order given*. The groups of continuities are specifically designed to provide a balanced and flowing practice.

The meditation period in the majority of yoga classes is actually a misnomer. Anyone familiar with the practice knows that meditation is silent and can only be entered when the body is relaxed and the mind is quiet and able to concentrate. This is why I have chosen to name this section "Relaxation/Meditation."

Few students will come to yoga with experience in meditation. It is important that you first learn the correct ways to relax your body, quiet your mind, and direct your concentration. This book addresses the need to learn a variety of ways in which to relax and become aware of your own energy. The book's Relaxation/Meditation sections progress through various visualization techniques that will allow you to increase your awareness. Finally, as a truly advanced student, you will experience light, love, and universal energy. Always practice the Relaxation/Meditation lesson that you feel is most appropriate for the present moment in your journey.

You might want to read aloud and record the Relaxation/Meditation ahead of time, so that you can fully experience the meditation. These sections include appropriate places for you to pause and experience certain aspects of the practice. As you record yourself, speak slowly and always keep your voice low, soothing, and caressing. Remember that when you listen to yourself again, you will be in a deeply relaxed state. Watch yourself for any signs of discomfort, distress, or tension. If this occurs, gently guide your thoughts back to your breath.

For those of you who are teachers, I hope you will find this book useful as a guide for building your classes and guiding your students. Feel free to adapt the meditations at the end of each lesson to your own classroom. Keep in mind that new students come to class because they are looking for something. It is the teacher's responsibility to help these students find whatever it is they seek. The teacher acts as a guide who points the way and presents knowledge. It is not the teacher's responsibility to impose his or her own beliefs and practices upon others. A teacher is merely a conduit. Ultimately, it is up to the individual student to decide whether or not to continue to grow in the wisdom of yoga.

It is not the purpose of this book to give a lesson in Sanskrit—the language of the yogas. Therefore, I have chosen to refer to yoga postures by their standard, English names, which will be familiar to any yoga practitioner. What is far more important is that you gently learn how to move your body correctly; how and when to inhale; how and when to exhale; how to stretch, but not strain; how to use, but not abuse.

Yoga is a gradual process, and progress is as individual as each student. Generally, taking a week to go through each lesson, practicing the postures once a day, will bring you the most benefit. Do not to attempt more advanced postures until you have developed the appropriate level of flexibility. It is important that you learn the correct breathing techniques that will relax your body before attempting any of the postures.

Your goal should not be to quickly progress in a particular posture, but to get the most out of what and where you are now. Awareness and attitude are what count. Bringing your body, mind, and breath into balance will bring balance and harmony into your life. I don't want you to be better than someone else. I want you to be the best that you can be.

The postures outlined in this book are not necessarily difficult to practice. However, if you find yourself struggling with any of the postures, don't try to exceed the limits of your own body. Your body will tell you how far you should move into a posture. Learn to relax *into* the posture and breathe properly while doing it. Above all, think positively; tell yourself that you can do it. Keep in mind that often those who find greater difficulties also find greater meaning. Whenever you think that a posture is difficult and that you can't do it, simply close your eyes and very slowly picture your body performing it absolutely perfectly. Then, try it again. Once you visualize yourself in the posture, your body will follow through.

How long should you hold each posture? Some days you may only want to hold the Plow position for thirty seconds, if you're not in the mood. On other days you might want to stay in position for five minutes. You should hold each posture for as long as you find it comfortable and your body tells you that it wants and needs to stay there. If you are uncomfortable in any posture, simply come out of it right away. There are no benefits to staying in a position that is uncomfortable. When you first learn postures, you should try to hold them at least ten seconds. As you become more advanced in your practice, you'll want to follow your mind: Only hold the posture if it is comfortable.

A good way of testing your body for weakness is to enter a particular posture and hold it longer than you usually would. The part of your body that becomes tired or sore is the weakest part of your body— the part you want to take care of. If you want to find out how much stress your body retains, do a Neck Roll before you begin your postures. Do you hear all that sand scratching around? You can measure your stress level by the amount of noise your neck makes. Try practicing the Neck Roll again at the end of your practice. If you have done your postures correctly—aware of each movement and each breath—the scratching sound should be reduced. Yoga is the essence of relaxation and the best stress remedy you will ever take.

Remember that living should be fun. Life should be a joy. Students who experience inner peace and harmony through yoga practice learn to carry this joy into their daily lives. So, if you are ready, let's discover YOU!

Shanti—Shanti—Shanti

Beginner Level Lessons

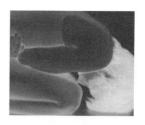

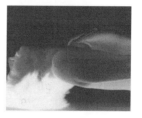

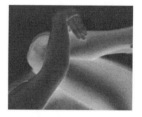

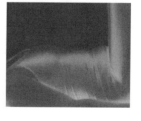

BEGINNER LEVEL LESSON 1

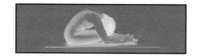

Proper breathing, perhaps the most important part of yoga, results in better health, sounder sleep, less disease, a clearer mind, and more cheerfulness. It slows the aging process and helps us feel light and supple. With yoga, we achieve perfect circulation. We relieve backaches, arthritis, bursitis, and headaches. We no longer feel tired, overweight, or underweight. With proper breathing, we can learn how to cool ourselves, how to warm ourselves, how to energize ourselves, and how to calm ourselves.

The Importance of Breathing

Our body removes 3 percent of its waste through the bowel, 7 percent through urine, 20 percent through our skin, and 70 percent by breathing. In yoga, relaxation is the "art," beathing is the "science." Here are some of the most important reasons why we need to maximize our breathing capacity:

1. The tempo of our respiration determines all our body/mind activities. Although we breathe approximately 23,000 times a day, we do so on automatic pilot and don't think about breathing properly. Yoga brings our attention to breathing properly.

2. Most of us use only one-sixth of our lung capacity, which causes us to become tired. Oxygen is fuel for our body. Our body renews itself twelve times a year, chiefly through oxygen, or what yoga calls prana energy, not through food.

3. Our brain needs three times more oxygen than the rest of our body. We can't digest our food without oxygen. We also need oxygen to break down food molecules and convert them into energy.

4. Inadequate oxygen speeds aging.

5. All organs suffer without proper oxygen.

6. People who suffer from cancer have an oxygen deficiency.

7. A lack of oxygen can cause tension, sleeplessness, constipation, nervous headaches, heart conditions, and mental disabilities.

8. We can literally, *literally*, breathe away ills, tension, and fatigue if we breathe properly.

9. Yoga postures are much easier to perform with proper breathing. We *inhale* to lift our body, and we *exhale* to bring our body back together.

10. Proper breathing is the doorway to meditation.

How to Approach Your Yoga Practice

When you begin to practice your postures, simply sit for a moment. Breathe deeply, make sure your body is totally relaxed and free of stress. This will allow you to perform the postures more easily and without hurting yourself. Make sure to wear loose clothing so that your body is free to move. You should wait three to four hours after having a large meal, one to two hours if you have had a light snack, such as a sandwich, and at least one half hour if you have had liquids.

The best time to practice is early in the morning. Why? It keeps us from putting it off until the afternoon or the evening, when something is likely to come up, or we might feel like watching television instead. In the morning, our stomach is already empty, so we don't have to worry about waiting for any food to digest. We are also less likely to be interrupted. It's best not to start if you are going to be interrupted, if you have to worry about children or the phone ringing. Besides, practicing yoga first thing in the morning truly sets the pace for our entire day. We have stretched our body into aliveness; it feels good and is ready to move. We sit for a moment and breathe deeply. Our mind is at peace, and we can go out and take on whatever the day throws at us.

Let me give you one last thought before you begin your postures. Yoga has been delicately, deliberately, and decisively formulated to allow us to become masters of our own senses, rather than being slaves to them. It allows us to enjoy a healthier physical life and a more peaceful mental life. It even allows us to become acquainted with our spiritual side. Yoga brings all these aspects into balance and harmony in a most gentle way. And, perhaps best of all, we get to meet a very special person—our real self.

Remember, the rule in yoga is this: you are not in a competition. Each body is different. Perform each posture only to the extent that your body will allow, not what someone else can do. Listen to your body. Our body whispers to us all the time, but we don't listen. We wait for it to scream and, then, it's generally too late.

Now, let's get healthy together.

Postures

1. Dreaming Dog.

Lie on the floor on your back with your arms by your sides, and very gently bounce your arms and legs up and down, like a dog having a dream and ''running'' while asleep. This will get your circulation flowing very gently through your body.

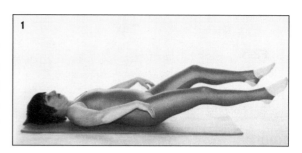

2. Lie and Stretch.

Lie on the floor just as in Dreaming Dog. Inhale and lift your arms over your head. Stretch your legs forward, as if you were just waking up. Really stretch your body. You want to get your circulation to go up and down your spine, moving within the negative and the positive, the yin and the yang.

Rotate your wrists and ankles as you stretch. Really stretch, then exhale and relax.

3. Leg Raise I and II.

Lie on the floor with your arms at your sides. Inhale and lift one leg straight up. Exhale slowly and lower your leg to the floor. Repeat this movement with your other leg, inhaling to lift and exhaling to lower. Then, inhale and lift both legs up. Exhale very slowly and lower your legs to the floor. This posture is very good for your stomach muscles.

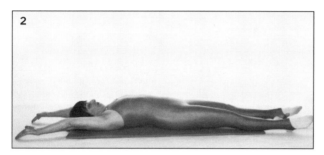

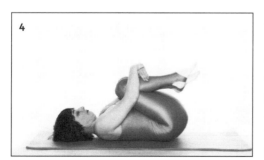

4. Reverse Bow I and II.

Lie on the floor, inhale, and lift one leg. Bend it at the knee and clasp it with your arms. Exhale and bring it toward your chest, while keeping your other leg flat on the floor. Inhale, release your leg and return it to the straight up position. Exhale and lower it to the floor. Repeat this movement with your other leg. Inhale to lift it, and clasp it with your arms. Exhale to bring it to your chest. Inhale to lift it straight up, and exhale to lower it to the floor. Repeat this movement with both legs at once. Inhale to lift them, and wrap your arms around them. Exhale to bring your legs to your chest. Inhale to lift them straight up, and exhale to lower your legs very slowly to the floor. This posture is excellent for your stomach muscles and for relieving your lower back area.

5. Fish.

Lie on the floor and raise your upper body with your elbows. Lean your head back so that the top of it is on the floor. Release your elbows and stretch your arms out, along your thighs. Breathe normally. To release the posture, return your elbows to the bent position at your sides, gently lift your head out of the

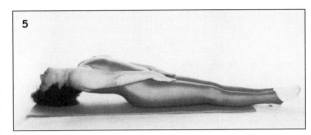

position, and slowly lower your upper body back to the floor. When your head is tipped back on the floor, you should feel a tightness in the neck area; then, you know it's working.

This movement allows you to open up your chest cavity and is good for bronchial and lung ailments. The Fish pose also helps stimulate the thyroid, parathyroid, and pituitary glands. It corrects posture problems, alleviates stiffness in the spine, and relaxes and beautifies the neck. The Fish is also effective for regulating the bowels, menstruation, and relieving hemorrhoids. Further along in your practice, you should use it to open your chest back up after compressing it with the Shoulder Stand.

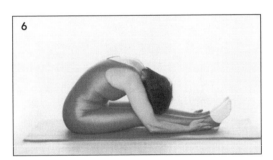

6. Head to Knee and Pull.

Lying on the floor with your legs straight, inhale and raise your arms over your head. As you begin to sit up, hold your breath. Exhale as you bend forward and bring your body together, resting your head on your knees. Grab your toes, hold on to them, and try to look up at the ceiling. This posture nicely stretches your back area.

7. Neck Roll.

Sit in a cross-legged position on the floor. Relax your neck, pointing your chin to your chest. Inhale, roll your head to your right shoulder; then, roll it toward your back. Exhale to roll it to your left shoulder.

Relax your chin down to your chest again. Repeat this roll three times for each side. If you feel dizzy after each rotation, simply turn a half circle in the opposite direction, and the dizziness will disappear. As you roll your neck, you will probably hear sounds like grains of sand. The louder the noise, the more stress and tension are in your body. This posture is excellent for relaxing your neck area and for relieving headaches. If you have, or have had, neck injuries or discomfort, you may wish to return your neck to a center position between each movement.

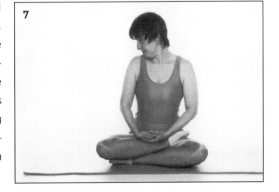

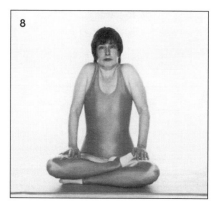

8. Shoulder Lift and Roll.

Sit in a cross-legged position on the floor. Inhale and lift your shoulders up toward your ears. Exhale and let them drop down. As you practice this posture, sigh on the exhalation. Your body enjoys the "sigh," which tells it to relax. Repeat the pose three or four times, inhaling up and exhaling down. Then, roll your shoulders in a backward motion three or four times and forward three or four times. This posture releases the tension in your body, and relieves you of stress, fatigue, neck ache, and headaches.

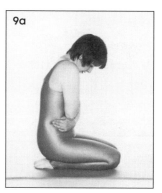
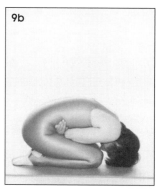

9. Elimination.

This posture's name indicates its purpose. From a kneeling position, sit back on your heels. As you inhale, lift your arms and cross them in front of your body in the area between your lower rib cage and slightly above your hip bone. Exhale, bend forward, and rest the top of your head on the floor, while keeping your buttocks on your heels. Rest in this position for three to four minutes. You should feel a lot of movement in your stomach area. If you don't feel a change taking place, inhale, gently rise out of the position, and drink a glass of warm water. When you return to the position, you should feel movement in your stomach. It's preferable to perform this posture first thing in the morning when your body is empty. Do not practice this pose on a full stomach; it would be very uncomfortable.

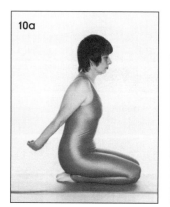
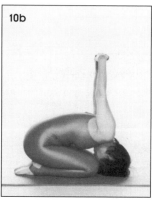

10. Kneeling Reverse Arm Raise.

Sit with your buttocks resting on your heels. Inhale, bring your arms behind you, and clasp your hands together. Exhale and lower your body forward, with your face to the floor. On the exhalation, raise your arms behind you as high as you can, leaving your buttocks on your heels. You'll want to feel the pull in your shoulders. Release your hands and, as you inhale and lift your body, let your arms fall to your sides. This posture releases stress in your shoulder area.

11. Lion.

Kneel as in the previous pose. Rest your hands on your knees, close your eyes, and inhale deeply. As you exhale, push your tongue out forcefully and try to reach down to the bottom of your chin. Open your eyes wide, extend your fingers, and push your palms into your knees. You may feel a little odd practicing this posture for the first time. However, when you realize that simply pushing your tongue out will prevent or relieve a sore throat, then you won't feel so silly. The Lion pose does this by stimulating circulation to your throat and tongue. This posture is also very good for your facial muscles.

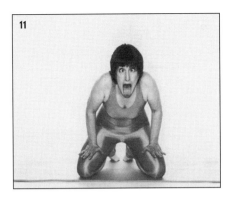

12. Sitting Spinal Twist.

If you have had back surgery, you should refrain from performing this posture. Start by kneeling and resting your buttocks on your feet. Then, let your buttocks slide to the right side and down to the floor. Bring your left leg up, bending it at the knee. Place your left foot on the outside of your right knee. Hold your left foot with your right hand. Inhale and twist to the left, while placing your left arm behind you with your palm on the floor as close to your buttocks as possible. Try to see the wall behind you. Exhale and relax to the original forward position. Repeat this movement for the opposite of your body, trying to keep your buttocks on the floor and twisting only at the waist. This posture is excellent for keeping your spine in a supple condition. It massages your stomach, kidneys, liver, and pancreas. This twist alleviates constipation, indigestion, rheumatism, and sciatica. It has also been said to help emphysema patients.

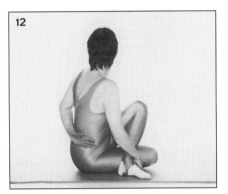

13. Standing Head to Knee.

Stand with your feet comfortably apart. Inhale and place your hands behind your back. Exhale and bend forward between your legs, with your arms raised upward behind you. Do not bend your knees. Inhale and twist to the right. Place your head to your right knee, and keep your arms raised behind you. Exhale. Inhale to lift your body, and lower your arms. Exhale and relax. Repeat this movement for the right side of your body; then, repeat down to the middle. This posture is good for your legs, and you'll feel the pull in the back of them. It also helps get circulation to your head, which is vitally important and should be practiced each day. Poor circulation to the head results in decreased blood and oxygen to the brain, which may cause senility. This posture also keeps your pituitary gland supplied with plenty of oxygen.

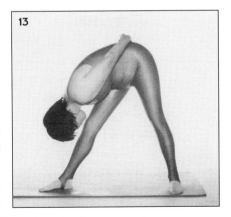

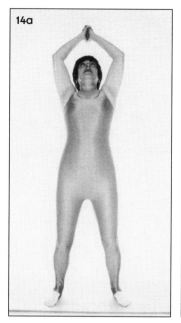

14a

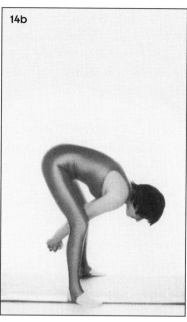

14b

14. Wood Chop.

Stand with your legs apart, and imagine that there is a log about knee-high in front of you. Inhale and raise your head and arms as though you were clasping a heavy axe. Exhale as you vigorously try to bring your imaginary axe down and chop the piece of wood in half. As soon as you "strike the log," let your arms hang loosely, and release forceful outward breaths. This action cleanses your lungs. Let your torso swing naturally, three to four times, and let it stop naturally. Pause and relax. Inhale and raise your torso again.

Relaxation/Meditation: Complete Relaxation 1

Just as there is a right way and a wrong way of doing our postures, there is a right and wrong way of relaxing. We often think that to relax, all we need to do is to lie down, but we don't think about how we lie down. Most of the time, we are far from having placed our body in a properly relaxed state. Unconsciously, we still hold back by being uptight and tense. Had we the consciousness of an animal — a dog for example—then, indeed, we could just lie down. If you witness a dog's entrance into relaxation, you'll notice how, after having played or exercised its body, it simply flops to the floor, completely uninhibited, loose, limp, released, and relaxed. The dog is truly in the moment, in the act, naturally and unthinkingly complete. Not so for us. We truly don't know how to "let go." We carry the tightness and tension of the day with us, even when we lie down to the very relaxation we crave. We certainly knew how to relax when we were babies. Feel how a baby's body rests in your arms, totally relaxed. Unfortunately, we lose that trust in relaxation, that "letting go," as we grow older and "uptight." We must re-learn or, in truth, un-learn. We must go back and recapture what we have lost, but desperately need.

How Are You Breathing?

One reason for our being unable to relax properly and thoroughly is our inadequate breathing. Our breath is so shallow, so limited, so incomplete that it is a wonder we stay alive and make it through the day. We think of our lungs as "them." "As long as I get a little air in them, I'll be O.K." Of course you will, for a while. So will your car if you just run it on one cylinder, but, be assured, a breakdown is on the way. We think that if we lift our shoulders and suck in our stomachs, we have inhaled deeply. This is equally wrong. We have done nothing. Think of that dog I mentioned. It inhales by expanding its stomach and exhales by letting it fall. That, too, should be our way of proper breathing. Picture your abdomen as a balloon. As it fills up, it expands, and it empties as it collapses. The intake of oxygen, or what yoga calls prana energy, should not be limited to just the nostrils. The energy should continue to the larynx and to the windpipe, subdivide at the bronchial tubes, and subdivide again at the air sacs. When your breath is released, you should feel your abdomen deflate, the air pass upward through your body and out of your nostrils. Try this now.

Lie down, and without thinking about it, simply become aware of your breath by placing your hand on your abdomen. Inhale and feel it fill up. As you exhale, your abdomen will naturally lower itself again. It is all very natural, regardless of whether you are sitting, standing, or doing something else.

Lying Down Properly

As mentioned previously, there is a proper way to lie down—a good way. From your sitting position, simply stretch your legs out in front of you, keeping them close together, with your heels touching. Keep your eyes on the space between your two big toes. Slowly lie back by following an imaginary line all the way down to the floor. By imagining this line, you bring your body to rest on the floor in an evenly balanced manner—not to one side or the other—with your head aligned with your spine. This is important because your energy needs to flow in a smooth, even fashion through your body. We all have a weak side and a strong side to our body. We unconsciously have the habit of humoring our weakest side by not lying on it. As a result, over a period of time, the weak side becomes weaker. The idea of yoga is to bring your body into harmony, into perfect balance. Each side of your body must be treated equally, whether moving or resting, in order to keep this perfect balance.

After reclining your body, by following your imaginary line from your big toes to the top of your head, it is very advantageous to say to yourself: "Relax! I am going to *truly* relax. This is *my* time to just let go and to just *BE*!" And then, do it, and let your breath help you.

While inhalation is great for energy, it is your exhalation that helps you to let go and relax. As you lie down, concentrate on your exhalation and, with each new exhalation, let yourself go deeper and deeper into relaxation. Think about sinking into a feather bed. Concentrate not only on your outer body, but your inner body as well. Make sure that you relax every muscle, every ligament, every tendon. This is not an easy task for a beginner. Most of us are so used to holding back or up, rather than sinking down and in. Simply try it. It's definitely worth the effort. You might discover, maybe for the first time, how good it feels to be completely relaxed. Really feel it and really experience it. Become one with it.

Simply lie there, and become used to the idea that it's okay to "just be." Not only is it okay, but it is vitally important to your well-being. Just as your body needs movement, your mind needs rest, and your spirit needs inspiration. You must consider and take care of all three aspects of yourself, if you truly wish to become a whole, healthy, and happy person. By just following your breath, you are resting your mind. When you rest your mind, you can take better care of your body, for the mind dictates the body. If your mind is tired, it cannot do the kind of job it should do, and it cheats your body. I call it "push and pause." "Push," in the sense that we use our body by stretching it and strengthening it.

"Pause," in the sense that we rest our mind. The "pause" is just as important as the "push," so don't ignore it.

This first lesson in relaxation is a way of getting acquainted with the "you" that you might have been ignoring for a long, long time. Most of us take ourselves for granted until we finally reach a point where we have to become determined to do something to get our lives back together again. We want to live, not just exist.

When you are ready to come out of this rest time, instead of concentrating on your exhalation (the letting go), concentrate on your inhalation. Feel the energy fill you, and feel more alive, becoming more aware of your surroundings. Stretch, ever so gently at first. Then, finish with a really full stretch and yawn. You might want to twist, lift your legs, or do whatever your body feels like doing at this moment. As you are doing this, keep in mind this affirmation: "My body is relaxed and my mind is peaceful." Keep repeating it, and it might make you want to smile. Then, go ahead and smile. Smiling also heals your body and your mind.

We have learned more about our breath—to breathe more deeply, more fully, slowly—and we have learned how to recline the body to give it the best potential to come into balance and harmony. That's a big step, but so are most first steps into something we are not familiar with. But be assured, this step is one in the right direction for you.

We follow the dictates of the mind and ignore our intuitions.
It is the whispering of the heart that leads us to wisdom.
Shanti—Shanti—Shanti—Peace—Peace—Peace

BEGINNER LEVEL LESSON 2

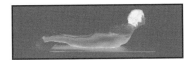

As you learned in the first lesson, breathing is very important. Every time you inhale, you should feel your abdomen expand and inflate like a balloon. We sometimes find it difficult to experience the rise and fall of the abdomen while standing or sitting. When you go to bed tonight, place your hand on your abdomen and notice that when you inhale your abdomen rises and that when you exhale, it falls. Your goal is to breathe normally, naturally. Our body produces three billion cells a minute. Not a single cell can be built without red blood, and no red blood cell can be built without oxygen. So, if you want to keep your cells happy and yourself happy, breathe deeply.

Prana Energy

We can survive sixty to ninety days without food, twelve to fifteen days without water, but only four to five minutes without air—prana energy. When we breathe, we should try to exhale twice as much as we inhale. For example, if you're inhaling to the count of four seconds—one, two, three, four—you should try to exhale to the count of eight seconds. However, you shouldn't turn purple trying. This is just a goal to aim for. If you can only exhale to six or seven seconds, that's okay, too. In time, you will build up your capacity for breathing, and your inhale/exhale count will increase from five to ten, six to twelve, etc. When you become comfortable in learning to exhale twice as much as you inhale, then you'll start to hold your breath in between your inhalation and your exhalation. In other words, if you are inhaling to the count of four and exhaling to the count of eight, you will hold your breath for a count of sixteen between your inhalation and your exhalation. Thus, your breathing count becomes: inhale for four seconds, hold for sixteen seconds, and exhale for eight seconds. The count for an inhalation of five seconds and exhalation of ten seconds is: inhale for five seconds, hold for twenty seconds, and exhale for ten seconds. As you become more advanced, you can increase your counts accordingly. But always remember to build up your count gradually. Don't force it yourself, but let it come naturally. In time, you will learn to breathe more deeply.

Nutrition

After a couple of weeks of yoga practice most people feel a lot better, both physically and mentally.

However, some become tired. If you have been lethargic, not exercising much and not breathing deeply, and you begin practicing postures or doing any exercise, your system begins to release toxins. This is actually a *good* sign because it shows that your body is beginning to cleanse itself. In order to help your body flush out these toxins, you should drink plenty of water. Be grateful that you are cleansing your body. Drink your water!

Now, let's talk a little bit about food. I'm not going to tell you what to eat. I'm going to give you some suggestions, and the rest is completely up to you. Yoga classifies food in three groups: sattvic, rajasic, and tamasic. Sattvic foods include fruits, vegetables, grains, nuts, and dairy products. These contain all the vitamins, minerals, amino acids, and enzymes necessary to control our metabolism. The true yogi or yogini only eats these calm, nourishing, and pure foods.

The average person eats sattvic foods as well as rajasic foods, which are spices, sugar, fried foods, coffee, and tea. This type of food is active, or stimulating, and may cause pain and disease. Fried foods are hard to digest, and could cause constipation. Certainly, the saturated fat from frying is known to clog arteries, giving us high cholesterol and heart attacks. Sugar causes a lack of energy after the initial boost, and gives some of us the discomfort of diabetes. Sugar interferes with digestion, making us feel bloated and sometimes instigating acid reflux. Coffee and tea are stimulants that contain caffeine, and overuse can lead to depression. Spices disturb meditation, because after a spicy meal, we are not calm.

Tamasic foods and substances are toxic to the body and stagnate the mind. They include meat, liquor, drugs, tobacco, overcooked food, and spoiled food.

The transition to pure, natural foods should be made slowly; otherwise the change to your system is too drastic. Those of us who eat pure foods would probably feel ill if we decided to eat at a fast food restaurant. It's too much of a change for the body to suddenly handle. However, you might want to consider gradually changing your diet to pure, natural, healthy foods.

One of the first foods you consider eliminating is meat. This, of course, is your decision. Yoga practitioners have known about the effects that meat has on the body for a long time. We will go into further detail on how to make dietary transitions in the next lesson. For now, I just want you to think about what you are eating.

In the Bible, we read that Methuselah lived nine hundred years. Genesis 1:29 states: "Every herb bearing seed and every tree in which is the fruit of a tree yielding seed to you they shall be for meat." In the beginning, people didn't eat meat until the flood came. Then, they began to eat meat in order to sustain themselves. Later, they forgot to give it up again, and from that point on, we just didn't live nine hundred years, did we? Although we may not be interested in living nine hundred years, we still want the years we do live to be healthy, so we can enjoy life.

The American Medical Association has also begun to consider the dangers of meat consumption. Hardening of the arteries, heart ailments, cancer, and other diseases have been linked to eating meat, especially red meat, which contains uric acid. Cell destruction is due to high blood acidity caused by an excess of acid-forming animal protein. When animals are led to the slaughter house, you can see the panic and fear in their eyes. This intense fear causes a great deal of toxins, including uric acid, to flow into their system. Regardless of how much the meat is "cleansed," this uric acid cannot be taken out of the animal. This is what we eat if we eat meat. Our liver and kidneys can extract only six grams of uric acid a day; the rest remains as poison in our systems. A pound of liver contains nineteen grams of uric acid, while a pound of beef steak contains fourteen. Since our liver and kidneys can only clear out six grams, the rest turns to gout, headaches, convulsions, nervousness, hardening of the arteries, heart attacks, and cancer. White blood cells always increase after a meat meal because these cells are fighting the toxemia caused by eating meat. In some people, the white blood cells don't stop producing, which is the cause of leukemia. Schizophrenia can also result from protein toxemia.

People sometimes say: "Well, if I can't eat meat, how am I going to get my protein? Protein is very important." Of course it is, but we don't need as much as we were taught we needed back in the early to mid-1900s, when most of us had jobs that involved heavy physical labor. Furthermore, you do not need putrefied protein from meat. Your body wants pure protein. For instance, nine almonds a day will give you all the protein that your body needs. Soy beans are also full of protein.

Did you ever go to a supermarket and see meat looking nice, red, and fresh in the meat case? Well, that's red dye, hiding the true state of the meat's putrefaction. In addition, animal feed is grown and treated with pesticides, while the animals themselves are fed growth hormones, antibiotics, and tranquilizers. In some instances, animal feed also contains processed meat from dead and diseased animals. A few years ago, in the wake of "Mad Cow Disease," government officials discovered that some cow feed contained meal made of dead and diseased cows and that sheep were being fed meal made from dead and diseased sheep. Cattle and sheep are ruminants, which means that they should only eat grass. Unfortunately, the industry's greediness is often the cause for these inhumane conditions. If we consume meat, we also consume these toxins. Dogs and cats are beginning to get our illnesses because their food is subjected to the same preparation as ours.

White flour turns to sugar in our liver, and should be avoided as well. And if you need a good reason to cut down on salt and spices, simply keep in mind that Egyptians used to embalm dead bodies with them. Interestingly enough, when we begin to change our diet, we need less sleep and have more time to do other things. Those who eat cooked or mixed diets need eight to twelve hours of sleep; those who eat raw foods or those who are vegetarians only need three to six hours of sleep a night; fruitarians, God bless them, only need one to four hours sleep. Our bodies use sleep for repair, so the less toxins we ingest, the less damage we do to ourselves, and the need for sleep decreases. Digestion itself is work for the body. So food that is easier to digest makes it easier for our bodies to recover.

Another thought on food: the strongest animals, the absolute strongest animals, like the ox, the elephant, and the horse, are vegetarians.

When I began practicing yoga, I was eating meat. After class my teacher used to say: "Well, you're all going to get a hamburger now." And, yes, we did. But, gradually, my desire changed and I found myself wanting only whole foods. I can get excited about eating a carrot or a head of lettuce. The students that continued to practice yoga with me automatically changed their eating habits. There is something inside of us that wants to live and wants to be healthy. Our body doesn't truly want meat. Interestingly enough, a friend of mine, who used to be a devoted meat eater, automatically lost the taste for meat when she became very ill with cancer. Our body always tells us what it needs. Our body desperately wants to be well and works hard to be well. Your blood cells truly care about you, but they need your help. Be a friend to your cells. Be a friend to yourself.

Postures to Review

Let's begin with some breathing. Lie on the floor and make sure that your body is comfortable. Inhale and push your stomach out. Exhale and feel all the tension of the day leave your body. Inhale again and exhale. Release your stress, your tightness, your irritation. Wiggle your toes and your fingers. Roll your head around to loosen your neck. Relax your shoulders. As your breathing becomes softer and slower, feel your entire body relax more and more. Rest and relax. Then start moving your body with your postures.

Review all postures from Beginners Lesson 1 (pp. 8–12), performing them in the order given, before trying the new postures.

 ## New Postures

15. Toes, Flat, Chair, Tree (see page 19).

The first three positions are for your leg muscles, and the last one is for balance. Balance positions calm us. In order to hold a balance position, focus your attention on a spot on the floor three feet in front of you, but don't think about maintaining your balance, simply focus on that spot.

Toes: In a standing position, inhale, rise up on your toes, and raise your arms above your head. As you exhale, bend your knees, and, still on your toes, lower yourself down to the floor. Inhale and return to an upright position. Exhale and lower your arms to your sides.

Flat: Again, in a standing position, inhale, and lift your arms above your head. As you exhale, bend your knees, and lower your body. Keep your feet flat on the floor and bring your arms parallel to the floor. Try to hold this position. Inhale to lift your body up to the original position. Exhale.

Chair: Stand with your feet flat on the floor. Lift one leg, bend it at the knee, and cross it over your other leg. Flex the leg that you are standing on, as though you were going to sit down in a chair. Return to a standing position and repeat for the other side of your body.

Tree: Stand with your feet flat on the floor. Raise one leg and place your foot on the inner thigh of your other leg. Your palms are together in front of the chest. Try to hold this position. Repeat this movement for your other leg.

16. The Cobras (Three Variations, see page 20).

Cobra positions are beneficial to the female reproductive organs and the menstrual cycle. They also relieve indigestion and constipation and help keep the spine limber. Because they gently stimulate the nervous system, they prevent obesity and insomnia.

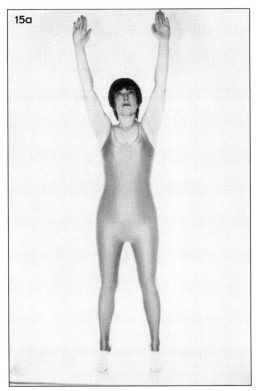

15a

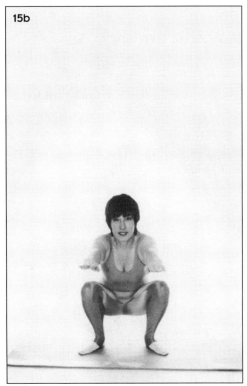

15b

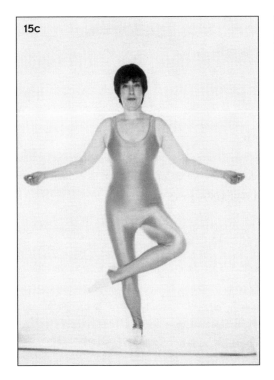

15c

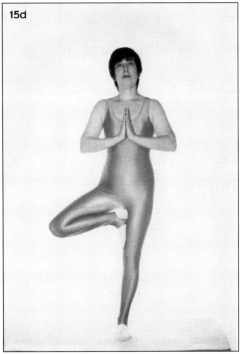

15d

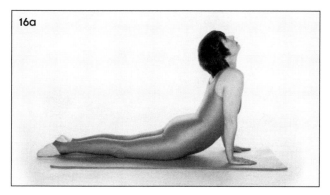

First Variation: Lie on your stomach. Place your hands on the floor right below your shoulders. Inhale and lift your head off the floor. Lift up each vertebra from your neck to your waist. Tilt your head back and look at the ceiling. Your arms are fully stretched. Try to hold this position. To lower your body, rest on your thighs, not on your knees, and exhale. Begin your exhalation at your waist and lower each vertebra to the floor. Your head should be the last thing to come down.

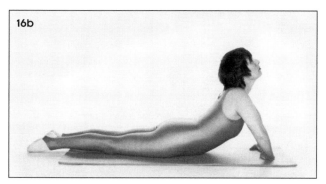

Second Variation: Lie on your stomach. Bend your elbows and place all your fingertips on the floor, under your chin and parallel to your body. Inhale and lift yourself like you did in the first variation. This time keep your elbows bent, rather than straight, and push your pelvic area into the floor, which will cause a greater curve to your back area. Exhale to lower your body, again, one vertebra at a time.

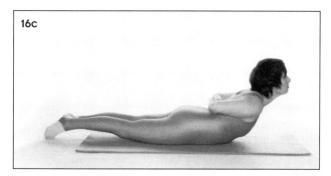

Third Variation: Lie on your stomach. Your hands may be at your sides or crossed behind your back. Inhale and lift the upper part of your body off the floor, starting with your head, and then each vertebra. Exhale to lower your body.

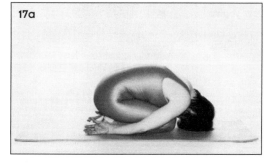

17. Infant Posture and Stretch.

This posture allows your spine to relax, and is an antidote for insomnia. It is also called the Sleeping Position.

Infant: Kneel and sit back on your heels, exhale, and lower your head to the floor in front of you. Your arms are relaxed with your palms facing the ceiling, along the sides of your body, like a baby sleeping. Hold this position, and simply think about relaxing each vertebra. It is particularly beneficial to do this posture after you have done the Cobras and other postures that place your spine in a similar curved position. This pose allows your spine to relax.

The Stretch: Begin from the Infant posture. Stretch, bring your arms up from your sides, and cross them in front of your head. Exhale and stretch one foot out behind you along the floor. Stretch your leg, as far as you can, out along the floor. Stretch, stretch, stretch. Then, relax into your extended side. Rest there for a moment. Inhale, bring your extended leg back to the Infant

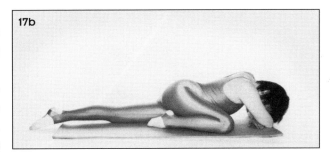

position, and stretch your other leg out, pushing your foot along the floor. Relax on that side, and rest for a moment. Inhale, bring your leg up, and lift your body to the kneeling position. You should feel very relaxed after this posture.

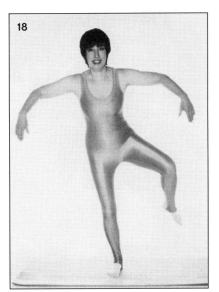

18. Skeleton.

Assume a relaxed standing position (don't lock your knees). Beginning at the top of your body, gently shake your shoulders up and down. Shake your arms. Shake your hands and fingers, as though you had water on them. While shaking your upper body, lift one leg and shake it out too. Alternate leg, and shake it out. This posture is very relaxing and beneficial to your circulation. It is also a good preparation for the standing postures.

19. Butterfly.

Sit on the floor. Bring your knees up and hold the bottoms of your feet together with your

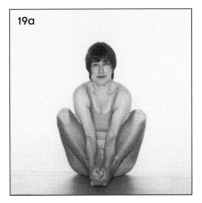

hands. Inhale and bring your knees up on the outside of your arms, as though you are giving them a hug. Exhale, let your knees fall out to the sides again, and drop them down. Try to reach the floor with them. Repeat this movement very slowly, up and down. Inhale to bring your knees up and give yourself a hug, and exhale to push them down to the floor. After you've practiced this gently for few times, you'll notice that it's almost like flying. Your knees are flying up and down, up and down, up and down. This posture loosens your hip joints and works your thighs as well.

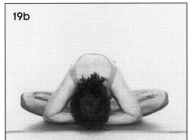

Advanced Butterfly: Remain in the Butterfly position, holding the soles of your feet together with your hands. As you hold your feet, push them slightly forward along the floor. Exhale, gently and slowly bend forward, and lower your head to your feet. Your arms should be on the outside of your legs. This movement stretches the vertebrae in your back. Inhale and return to an upright position.

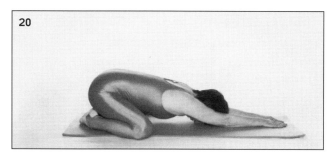

20. Forward Frog.

Kneel on the floor. Sit with your buttocks touching the floor between your heels and your toes touching behind you. Your knees are far apart in front of you. As you exhale, lower your body to the floor with your arms stretched out in front of you. Try to keep your buttocks close to the floor. Don't lift them up in the air. Try to hold this position. Inhale to lift your body up. This is a good stretch for your hips and inner thighs.

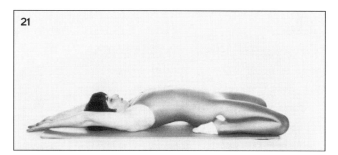

21. Reverse Frog.

Again, kneel on the floor, and sit between your heels with your buttocks touching the floor. Your legs are bent back and your feet are behind you. Lean back onto your elbows, and lower your body backward to the floor. Stretch your arms up and back onto the floor above your head. Again, you will feel the stretch in your thigh muscles.

When you are ready to come up, simply inhale to lift your body.

Relaxation/Meditation: Breathing Pain Away

Remember the imaginary center line that we used last week to lie down in a smooth motion on the floor. Make sure that your legs and feet are apart, at least to the width of your hips. Separate your arms slightly from the sides of your body. The palms of your hands should be facing upward. Once your body is properly aligned and comfortable, bring your attention to your head and neck. Is your head tipped back with your chin in the air? If so, simply lift up your head and gently place it down so that the back of your head is flat on the floor. This will relax your neck muscles and create less stress in your body. Neck pain can make your whole body feel uncomfortable, just as sore feet make your whole body feel tired.

Bring your attention to your face. Does it feel tight? Take a moment to think of something pleasant. Smile and relax the frowns. Tighten the area around your eyes and relax it. Wiggle your jaw and your mouth. Open your lips slightly and smile to yourself.

Concentrate on the exhalation of your breath, and remind yourself to become loose and limp, released and relaxed. Tell your body that it can let go; allow it to feel as if it is melting into the floor or into a feather bed. Really sink down and in. When you begin to let go, your body feels quite heavy. As you sink further down and relax more deeply, your body will feel lighter and lighter. You have set yourself free. You feel light, or might not have any awareness of your body at all. That is good!

Our bodies talk to us all the time. "My back is killing me"; "I've got a cramp in my leg." If your body is not whispering to you at this moment, then you've done everything right, and your body is grateful. If we learned to really listen to our bodies, we could take care of any problems when they are still mere whispers, when they are smaller and easier to solve. Unfortunately, we usually wait until our bodies are shouting at us and demanding that we pay attention. By then, the problem might be more serious and take longer to cure or correct. Sometimes, it might even be too late. So listen, heed.

Take a spot check of your body to make sure that you didn't miss anything. Is there tension anywhere? Is there pain? Is there discomfort? Take a moment to check your whole body. Give your arms and legs a slight wiggle. Check your back, your shoulders, and your neck. Don't miss any part of you. Move any part of your body that seems to need attention. If the tension doesn't respond to movement, try breathing it away.

There are three aspects to breathing away discomfort: 1) You must believe that you can do it; 2) You must think positively; 3) You must physically do it. Begin by concentrating on the area in need of assistance. For instance, if you feel tightness, picture the area relaxing as you exhale. Breathe the tightness away with your exhalation, and release it. If you feel pain, think the word "soft" around the area. Anytime that we feel pain, we unconsciously tighten up and are afraid to move. This tightness causes more tension, which causes more pain. But, if we picture the area growing soft, it will relax. This will help to reduce, relieve, or even eliminate the pain. Simply keep working on the area of discomfort until you breathe away the pain. You must know that you can do it. (Pause for a few minutes to practice this relaxation.)

Return to witnessing your breath: the inhalation, the pause, the exhalation. It is all very simple and very relaxing. The more you relax your breathing, the better your circulation will be throughout your body. Your body will feel renewed. Deep breathing relaxes and energizes us at the same time. This relationship is a good example of the perfect harmony of yin and yang—complementary opposites.

Pay attention to each inhalation and each exhalation. When you feel your breath passing in and out, you are participating in the movement of life. Now, stop regulating your breath in any way and simply follow it—the in and the out, the up and down, again and again, until there is no effort to your awareness, no effort to your movement, only a continual allowing and following and, finally, a beautiful becoming as of the breath itself. The dualistic aspect of "me" and the "breath" is gone! You have become the breath, or has the breath become you? The answer is not important. You feel light, suspended, calm, and free! You have truly let go, but you have also become. You now realize that this is relaxation. Smile. Smile not only on your lips but throughout your body. Rest in it for a moment or two, enjoying, basking, filling yourself with it, until the next time.

Once you are filled with this joyous feeling, gently bring your awareness back to the room around you, to your surroundings, to this moment. Begin to awaken your body back to aliveness. Begin with a very lazy stretch, then, stretch fully and yawn. You might want to twist, raise your legs, or do whatever your body tells you it needs at this moment. Listen! Then, do it!

One of the greatest gifts you can give yourself is the gift of silence.
It is there that truth will shout the loudest.
Shanti—Shanti—Shanti—Peace—Peace—Peace

BEGINNER LEVEL LESSON 3

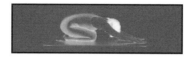

In the previous lesson, I talked about the three classifications of food and why a diet of sattvic food is best for us. In this lesson, I will talk about the foods that contain the important vitamins and minerals we need to keep ourselves feeling young. Three billion of our body cells die every minute, and in order to replace these cells, we need food rich in minerals and vitamins. Good food gives us fuel while minerals and vitamins help channel that fuel into body structure and strength.

Vitamins and Minerals

The most completely balanced food is whole grain brown rice. It contains five parts potassium, which is *yin*, or acidic, and one part sodium, which is *yang*, or alkaline. Yin expands and yang contracts. For example, sugar is yin. If you put sugar on your tongue, it expands. Salt, on the other hand, is yang. When you put salt on your tongue, it contracts. Anything that affects your mouth also affects your body, and, in turn, affects your mind. Neither yin nor yang is all good or bad; they are complementary opposites that should be in balance. Our goal shouldn't be to eat only brown rice. We should, however, eat a proper balance of food.

The B vitamins, found in high quantities in brewer's yeast, are good for digestive problems. Sugar robs our body of vitamin B. If you consume a lot of sugar, you should consider increasing your intake of vitamin B. We cannot survive without vitamin B. Although taking a multivitamin is a good start, it isn't enough for the average person. The addition of individual vitamins is more likely to better meet our body's requirements. A multivitamin will keep us functioning, but won't help us build good health. And isn't that the whole idea—to build health?

Why do we need to take vitamins at all? Our food is loaded with chemical fertilizers and pesticides, rarely grown organically. Consequently, it is robbed of the elements that occur naturally in unpolluted ground. Food is also kept in storage for long periods of time, which greatly diminishes its nutrient value. If you can catch an apple as it falls from the tree, or if you can grow your own organic vegetables and eat them immediately, you won't need additional vitamin and mineral supplements.

We destroy vitamins and minerals in the way we prepare our food. Take a single carrot, for example. Cutting the green top off depletes it of vitamin K. When we peel it, we lose its minerals. Soaking the carrot depletes it of its natural sugar, all B vitamins, most vitamin C, some vitamin P, and additional minerals. At this point, only calcium remains. If we decide to shred it, we lose 20 percent more vitamin C, and if we let it sit for a while, it will lose even more vitamin C. By adding salt, we lose whatever vitamin C was left to the carrot.

Processed foods are bleached, colored, dehydrated, hydrolized, homogenized, emulsified, pasteurized, gassed, preserved chemically, and canned. Obviously, we can't be getting many nutrients from these foods.

Bad habits destroy many of our vitamins. Smoking depletes us of vitamin C. Alcohol, coffee, and sweets deplete us of vitamin B. The chlorine in our water depletes vitamin E. Mineral oil destroys vitamins A, D, E, and K.

Vitamins control our body's appropriation of minerals. In the absence of vitamins, our system makes use of minerals. However, in the absence of minerals, vitamins are useless.

Dietary Recommendations

Heartburn is caused by hydrochloric acid and by sugar. Coffee with two teaspoons of sugar makes the mucous membranes in our stomach fiery red. It's like setting the stomach on fire the first thing in the morning. Sugar interferes with our digestion. When food can't be digested, we begin to feel bloated and take an antacid, which is the worst possible thing we can do. Antacids can cause calcium loss (which is why they now contain added calcium) and stop our digestive process completely, which results in constipation. If we're constipated, we take mineral oils, which in turn leach out vitamins and minerals from the body. It is truly a vicious and destructive cycle.

Nature's best remedy for gas or indigestion is garlic, which purifies our intestinal tract and acts as a digestive stimulant. Garlic is also a good cold remedy. Recently, it has been reported that garlic helps boost our immune system. And, in case you're worried about garlic breath, deodorized garlic is available.

We should try to eat our food at room temperature, neither too hot or too cold. These extremes are hard on our digestive system and contribute to arthritis. Fruits and vegetables, which are both excellent, should be eaten at least an hour apart. It takes a different digestive process for each one, and eating both in the same meal causes a conflict in our digestive system.

Our attitude while we eat is also very important. We shouldn't gobble our food, but savor each bite. We should try to simplify our meals. Eating many different types of food in one meal confuses our body and makes it work much harder. We should never eat more than three types of foods in one sitting.

Remember, you are what you eat! So the best foods are those that have the most energy in them—raw vegetables, fresh fruits—not those kept in storage for weeks and weeks. Most grains are easier to digest, and more filling and healthy than meat, fish, fowl, highly processed starches, and sugar. Don't think of your diet change as becoming vegetarian, think of it as your desire to be healthier, and live longer. Don't even change your diet all at once, or you'll feel deprived. Do it gradually, one thing at a time—just cutting down, not totally out—in the beginning. Start with only one serving of meat a day, then every other day, and so on. Soon, you won't miss it at all, and when you do eat it, you just won't feel as good. And, instead of carbonated drinks, try some fruit juices. In the beginning, add a little ginger ale or carbonated water to give the drink the "kick" you want. Try honey or maple syrup on your cereal—you'll get more energy from honey than you will from sugar. As for your proteins, there are two kinds: pure and putrefied. Pure has to do with nuts and beans and even some cheeses; putrefied means meat, which is toxic to the system. Meat may sound good to you, but if you start calling it what it really is—flesh—maybe it won't.

Postures to Review

It is time for you to lie down, to slowly and calmly breathe, and to pay attention to each inhalation and exhalation. Breathe away all your stress and tension. Relax your body. Release all your cares and stress. Inhale and exhale, and feel more and more relaxed. When you are ready, begin your postures.

Review all postures from Beginners Lesson 1 (pp. 8–12), performing them in the order given, before trying the new postures.

New Postures

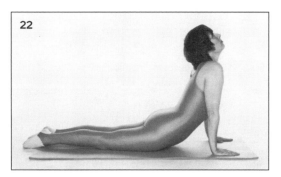

22. Swan.

Lie on your stomach with your hands on the floor under your shoulders. As you inhale, lift your body straight up as you did in Cobra (#16). Bend your knees, and raise your buttocks. Moving backward, slide your hands along the floor and relax back onto you heels. Your forehead should be close to the floor. To come out of this position, push your hands forward along the floor, as your nose moves along the floor. Raise your buttocks into the air, as your body follows your hands forward. At the full extension, inhale and lift your body up to Cobra position. Exhale and move backward again. Your arms are outstretched and your forehead is close to the floor. Rest. The final movement of the Swan posture looks almost like the movement of a snake. Originally, you moved straight up; then, you moved backward. However, when you push your hands forward, with your nose along the floor and your buttocks in the air, and as you move up and back a second time, your body is very curved and looks like a snake in motion.

23. Floating Swan.

This posture is generally performed after completing the Swan posture. Remain in the back-

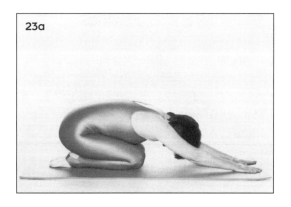

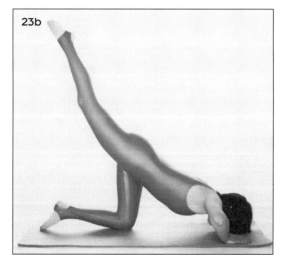

26

ward position of Swan, buttocks resting on your heels and arms outstretched in front of you. Bend your elbows and move your arms back slightly. Inhale and lift your body into a kneeling position, with your hands and knees on the floor. Slowly, as you exhale, keeping your back straight, lower your nose to the floor between your hands, and lift one leg straight up behind you. Try to keep your extended leg aligned with your back. Inhale and try to hold this position.

Exhale. As you lower your leg to the floor, your body rises and returns to a kneeling position. Inhale, lift your other leg, and lower your nose to the floor again. Exhale. As you lower your leg, your body rises, and you are back on all fours once more.

24. Balance on Fours.

In a kneeling position, with your hands and knees on the floor, inhale and lift your left arm and right leg until they are parallel to the floor. Hold the position. Exhale and lower down. Inhale and lift your right arm and left leg in the same manner. Keep your body straight, with your arms and legs out straight. Exhale and lower down. Next, inhale, lift your left arm and left leg and balance yourself. Exhale and lower down. Finally, inhale, lift your right arm and right leg. Hold the position, exhale, and lower down. Again, this is a very calming balance position.

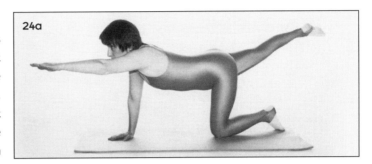

24a

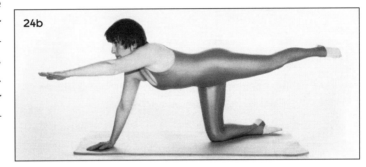

24b

25. Kiss the Foot.

Stand with your legs comfortably apart. Inhale, bring your hands behind your back, and clasp them. Turn your left leg and foot outward at an angle and bend your left knee. As you exhale, slide your right leg out to the side and lower your body down toward your left foot. You may raise your arms above you or hold them along your back, whichever is more comfortable for your balance. Inhale to raise your body. Repeat for the other side of your body. This posture stretches your legs. Again, the forward-downward movement brings circulation to your head.

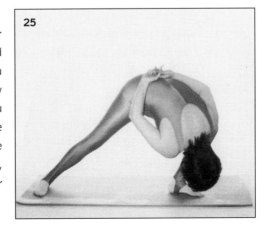

25

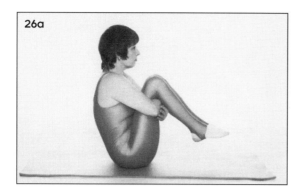

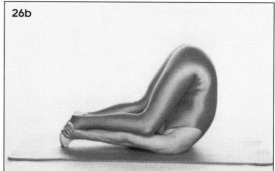

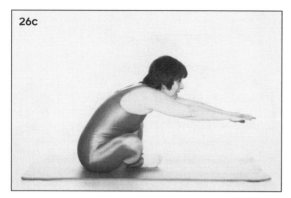

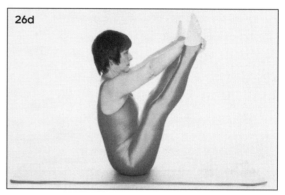

26. Full Rolls and Balance.

First Position: Sit on the floor with your knees raised. Clasp your hands together under your knees. Relax, truly relax. Roll backward with your feet coming over your head and try to touch the floor behind you. Again, be relaxed, and do not hold your body stiffly. Repeat four to five times and return to a sitting position.

Second Position: Still in a sitting position, move your arms to the insides of your legs, hold your ankles with your hands, and, again, roll backward. This time, as you roll forward, release your ankles and push your arms forward between your feet. Let the forward movement of your arms carry your body between your knees, and exhale vigorously. Repeat this movement four to five times. This posture helps to cleanse your lungs. While rolling backward and forward, remember how you felt as a child, rolling around on the floor, carefree.

Balance Position: After completing the second set of rolls, roll backward one more time. Roll forward and stop when you reach the upright position. Stretch your legs and arms up, balancing yourself on your buttocks, and hold your ankles with your hands. Again, the balance postures are very calming.

27. Sitting Leg Stretch Variations.

First Variation: Sit with your legs as far apart as possible. Inhale and raise your arms over your head. Exhale, bend forward, and place your chin on the floor between your feet. Let your hands reach for your feet. Inhale and raise your body to a sitting position.

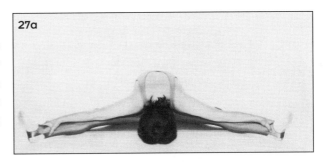

27a

Second Variation: Return to a sitting position. Exhale, turn to the right, and lower your body down toward your right leg, reaching for your right foot. Try to place your head on your right knee. Inhale and return to a sitting position. Exhale, turn your body to the left, and lower it down to your left knee, reaching for your left foot. Inhale and raise your body to a sitting position.

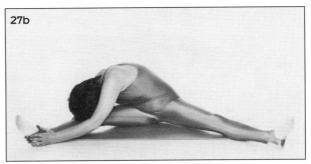

27b

Third Variation: From your sitting position, gently twist your waist to the left side. Exhale and lower your body down over your right leg. Slide your right arm down along your right leg, and stretch your left arm up over your left ear. Inhale and lift your body back to a sitting position. To repeat this movement for the other side of your body, gently twist your body sideways to the right at the waist, exhale, and lower yourself down over your left leg. Inhale and raise your body to a sitting position.

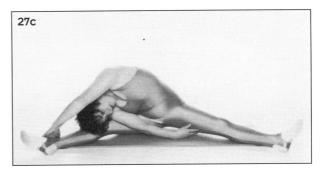

27c

Fourth Variation: After returning your body to a sitting position, extend your right leg forward, bring your left foot to the inside of your right thigh, and exhale down to your right leg. Try to place your head to your knee, reaching for your foot and grasping your ankle, or as close to your ankle as you can

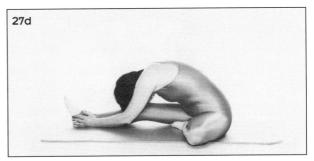

27d

reach comfortably. Inhale, as you raise your body to a sitting position, bring your right leg with you. Try to keep your knee close to your head. Exhale, lower your leg down very slowly, and let your body remain in a sitting position. Reverse these movements for the opposite side of your body. Extend your left leg and keep your right foot inside your left thigh. Lower your head down to your left knee, and raise and lower your left leg. Take a long, slow, relaxing breath. This posture stretches and twists your spine, and keeps it supple. All the movements should be very slow, smooth, flowing, and relaxed.

28. Cat Variations and Stretch.

First Variation: Kneeling on your hands and knees, with your palms on the floor and your fingers facing each other, inhale and arch your back up and down, up and down, very slowly. This movement strengthens your lower lumbar area and is very good for people with back problems.

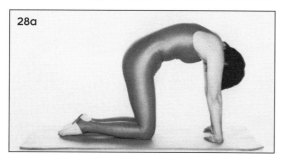

28a

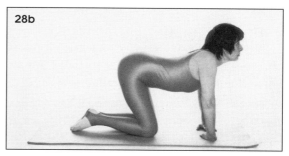

28b

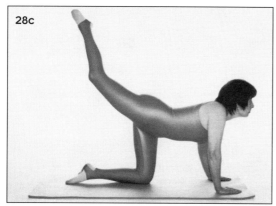

28c

Second Variation: Cat Kick. Again, kneel on your hands and knees with your palms on the floor and your fingers facing straight ahead. Take one leg and kick it up behind you as high as you can. Arch your back up, bend your head down, and bring your knee back to your nose. Repeat this posture three to four times for each leg.

Third Variation: Cat Stretch One. After completing Cat Kick, stay on your knees. Fold your arms on the floor in front of you and rest your head down on your arms, with your buttocks in the air. This variation is your resting stretch.

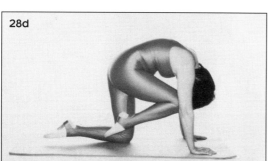

28d

Fourth Variation: Cat Stretch Two. After completing Cat Stretch One, push your arms straight out in front of you, as far as you can. Keep your nose to the floor and your buttocks in the air. You will feel a nice stretch in your shoulder area. Hold this posture for as long as it is comfortable. Inhale and raise your body.

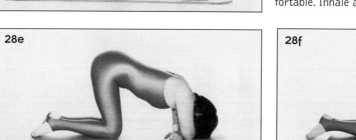

28e

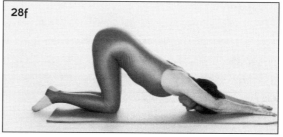

28f

Relaxation/Meditation: Listening for Silence

Begin this relaxation period by comfortably sitting for a few moments. Close your eyes and regulate your breath slowly in and out. Feel your stomach rise, as you inhale, and return inward, as you exhale. Your breathing should be rhythmic, not forceful. Always try to exhale twice as long as you inhale. This point is particularly important as you try to relax. Your outward breath is a good way to tell your body that it's alright to relax; it's alright to let go, to feel at peace.

As you first begin to learn to relax, to find your way into a meditative state of existence, silence becomes very important. Any noise can be a total distraction to your peace, to your success in reaching your goal of bliss. Because we pay so much attention to sound, we may miss hearing the silence altogether. Silence is a good way of tuning in to our self, the inner self that we fail to make contact with as often as we should. This relaxation will give you the opportunity to acquaint yourself with silence.

For a few minutes, with your eyes closed and your breathing relaxed to a smooth rhythm, try first to listen for silence. (Pause briefly to experience the silence.)

If you are having trouble tuning in, cover your ears with your hands. Take a few minutes and try to truly hear the silence. Try it now. (Brief pause.)

Now, stop. In addition to hearing the silence, you probably also heard you—your inner vibrations. Perhaps, you heard your heartbeat. You made contact, tuned in, touched base.

Lie down and adjust your body comfortably to the floor, balanced and centered in peace. Again, keep your eyes closed and give yourself permission to go loose and limp, released and relaxed. This time, instead of thinking about sinking into a feather bed, think about sinking into silence. Absorb it and let *it* absorb you. Do not let any outside thoughts enter your mind to disturb this blissful quiet, this serenity of silence. If a thought tries to come in, simply turn your attention back to your breathing. Breath in, breath out, and enter silence. Try it now. (Pause again.)

Know that all meaningful, miraculous things come in silence: the sunrise, the sunset, a breathtaking rainbow, a starry night, a look of love, a still pond, and, most importantly, your connection to your real self.

Rest a few more minutes, feeling completely relaxed. Feel the peace that surrounds you. Feel free and light. Feel rested but alive to this moment, this happening, this experiencing, this utter joy. Maybe realize for the very first time that the happiness we seek outwardly is already locked inside of us. We must be still, paused in the silence, to receive it. We must learn to trust ourselves to open up to the peace that is already ours. When we learn to let go, really let go, we will receive it. Only by emptying out, can we become filled, overrun with happiness.

Give yourself a positive thought to take with you. We become what we think, and every thought directs our life into what we become, into what we are. What will you be now?

Slowly, begin to stretch your body back to aliveness. Always start with your toes, then move your legs, your hands, and your arms into a gentle stretch. Finally, fully stretch into a yawn, and do whatever your body needs you to do before arising, maybe a turn or a twist. Let your final thought be: "Life is a celebration." Smile to yourself as you go back to your outer world.

When was the last time you let the seashell sing in your ear?

Held your face to the falling snow? Let a drifting flake rest upon your nose?

When was the last time you jumped into the center of a puddle?

Not over it?

Reached the palms of your hands out to gather the falling raindrops?

When was the last time you built sandcastles or wrote messages on the shore?

Or paused long enough on a summer day to allow the butterfly to land on your shoulder?

Well, what are you waiting for?

The experiencing of God may pass you by.

The clock ticks on. The calendar page is turning. Grasp this now

NOW!

Shanti—Shanti—Shanti—Peace—Peace—Peace

BEGINNER LEVEL LESSON 4

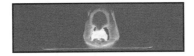

Yoga stretches and strengthens your body. However, you are more than just muscle and sinew. You are what you eat. In the last lesson, I briefly mentioned the importance of vitamins and minerals. Let's go over the important ones that you should pay attention to in your diet.

Essential Nutrients

Calcium builds bones and teeth. It calms nerves and aids insomnia. It is also helpful for rheumatic heart action. Calcium and iron need acid for simulation. If our body does not have enough acid, calcium begins to build up, which can lead to arthritis and bursitis. However, calcium combined with vitamin C (which is acidic) can relieve arthritis. Calcium also needs vitamin D for proper absorption.

Phosphorous works in combination with calcium. Although, our diets rarely lack phosphorous, if your body needs phosphorous, lecithin and brewer's yeast are both excellent sources. Brewer's yeast is also a good source of minerals, 13 B vitamins, and 16 amino acids. So keep that brewer's yeast handy!

Magnesium is missing from most peoples' diets. You can increase your magnesium intake by consuming nuts, whole grain products, dry beans, peas, soy products, and sea water.

Potassium aids our heart function and is absolutely essential to your health. A lack of potassium can upset your entire nervous system, lead to heart seizures, weak muscular control, and constipation. The best sources of potassium are raw foods, leafy greens, black strap molasses, and sunflower seeds.

Iodine is essential to our thyroid gland and stimulates energy. In excess, however, it can cause nervousness.

Iron gives us energy and promotes healthy breathing. It keeps our cheeks and lips pink and our eyes bright, and our zest for living to its fullest. Our red blood cells need iron.

Manganese, fluorides, sodium, chrome, zinc, and lithium are found in sea water in almost the same proportion as in our own blood stream. You can get all your minerals by eating kelp, either as a sea vegetable or as a tablet. It contains 22 minerals, plus trace elements. One kelp tablet about the size of an aspirin contains as much iron as 70 pounds of fresh fruit and vegetables, 56 pounds of grains and nuts, 12 pounds of eggs, or 2 pounds of fish.

Alfalfa is another rich source of minerals—with seven vitamins and six minerals—its roots grow very deep into the earth. You should try to drink hard water, which contains more minerals than soft water. Distilled water contains no minerals at all. Interestingly, it has been scientifically proven that both bursitis and arthritis respond to sea water. Have a good swim and have a good drink!

 ## Postures to Review

Gently lie back on the floor and breathe. Inhale and feel lightness enter your body. Exhale and feel all your tension and tightness being released. Inhale and feel light. Exhale and feel relaxed and released. When you are relaxed, begin your postures.

Review all postures from Beginners Lesson 1 (pp. 8–12), performing them in the order given, before trying the new postures.

 ## Postures

29. Camel.

Sit with your buttocks on your heels with your feet relaxed on the floor behind you. Inhale and place your hands on the floor behind your feet. Lift up your pelvic area and lean your head back. Try to hold this position. Exhale whenever you are ready to return to the opening position. This posture will stretch your thigh area.

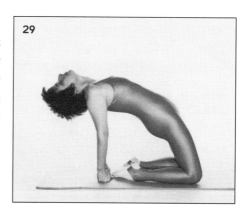

30. Standing Wall–Ceiling Stretch.

Standing with your feet comfortably apart, turn your left leg and foot outward, and turn your body to the left side. Bend your left knee and place your left hand on the outside of your left foot. Stretch your right leg out behind you, and stretch your right arm forward, as though you are trying to touch the wall in front of you. Inhale and stretch your right arm up to the ceiling. Don't just point up, truly stretch. Exhale and lower your arm behind you, with your palm facing up the ceiling. Turn your head and let your eyes follow the movement of your arm and hand. Rest in this position for as long as it is comfortable for you. Inhale, reach to the ceiling, and stretch to the wall in front of you. Return to a

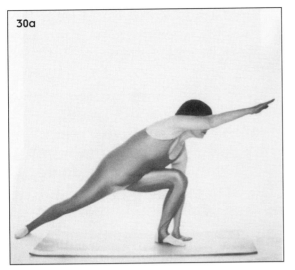

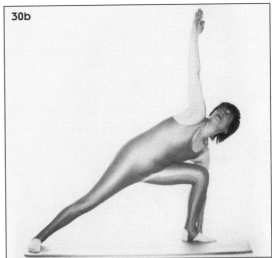

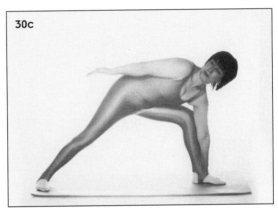

standing position. Repeat this rotation for the right side of your body. Turn your right leg out and your body to the left. Bend your right knee and place your right hand on the outside of your right foot. Reach out to the wall and up to the ceiling, and rest with your arm behind you and your palm up. Inhale, stretch your arm to the ceiling and to the front wall, and bring your body up to a standing position. Exhale and relax. This posture really stretches your body.

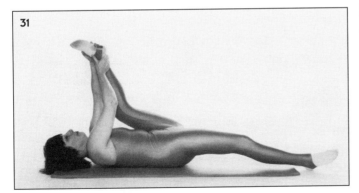

31. Lying Knee to Head.

Lie on the floor. Inhale and lift one leg up. Grab your toes with both hands and try to pull your foot behind your head, while keeping your other leg flat on the floor. Exhale and lower your raised leg very slowly down to the floor, releasing your toes as you lower your leg. Repeat this movement for the other side of your body. Inhale, lift your leg up, and grab your toes with both hands. Pull your foot behind your head as far as you can, and keep your other leg on the floor. Exhale and slowly lower your leg down. This posture stretches your hips.

32. Hare.

This is the first position in learning the Head Stand. Even if you never learn to master the Head Stand, Hare is a good position for getting circulation to the head. Assume a kneeling position. Bend forward onto your elbows and make your hands into fists. Bring your right fist to the inside of your left elbow and

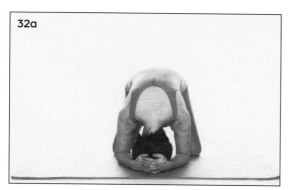

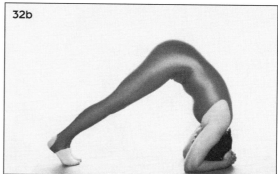

pivot your right fist forward, without moving your elbow. Bring your left fist to the inside of your right elbow and pivot your left fist forward, without moving your right elbow. Once in this position, which is your base, do not move your elbows. Without moving your elbows, open your fists, your palms facing you, and interlock your fingers, with your hands in an upright position. Place the top of your head on the floor with the back of your head touching the palms of your hands. Straighten your knees and lift your pelvic area up in the air so that your body forms an upside-down V. Rest in this position for as long as you feel comfortable. Very slowly, lower your knees to the floor and rest for a moment. Slowly, raise your head and your body up to a kneeling position.

33. Forward Boat.

Lie on your back. Inhale and lift your legs and torso upward. Stretch your arms forward on the outside of your knees. Your body will be in a V-shaped position balanced on your buttocks. Hold this position for as long as it is comfortable for you. Exhale and lower your arms and legs back to the floor. This is a good balance position that strengthens the body and calms the mind.

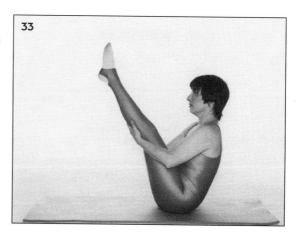

34. Ceiling Walk and Cross.

Lie on your back. Inhale and raise your arms and legs perpendicular to your torso. Take long, slow strides with your arms and legs, as if you were out for a walk on the ceiling. Move your arms and legs up and out, very slowly. If you want to rest, cross your arms and legs over each other and swing them from side

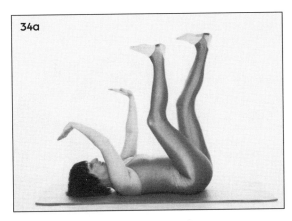

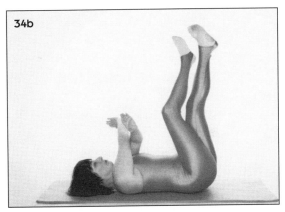

to side and back and forth. When you are rested, go for another walk across the ceiling. Come out of this position by lowering your arms and legs back to the floor. Take a slow relaxing breath.

35. Lying Knee to Floor.

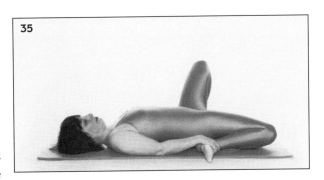

Lie on your back and bend your knees. Bring your heels as close to your buttocks as you can and grab your ankles with your hands Lower one knee inward toward the floor (your foot will roll over onto the instep), then bring it back up. Alternate this movement with each leg—first the right, then the left. This posture is particularly important because it loosens up the hip joints. Most people wake up in the morning with one leg longer than the other. It's not a good way to start the day. By taking a few moments each morning to practice this posture, you can get a better start to your day and have a lot less back pain.

Relaxation/Meditation: Deep Breathing

Before lying down into relaxation, acquaint yourself with some of the wonderful qualities of your breath. Your breath is a special friend, not only because it gives you life, but because you can call upon it to give you energy, to warm you, to cool you, to calm you, even to inform you. Let your breath inform you as to who and what you are. We all think we know who we are, but truly, we're only aware of the outer, everyday us, not the real being. Our breath reminds us of the real being every time we breathe in and breathe out.

Close your eyes and take a deep inhalation. (Brief pause.)

Slowly exhale. Do you hear anything? If you don't, try it again, and really listen this time. (Another brief pause.)

Slowly exhale. The sound that comes with the inhalation sounds like "so," coming in through the nostrils. Try it one more time and see if you can hear it now. (Brief pause.)

Pay attention to your exhalation. What sound does it make? Inhale and listen. (Brief pause.)

The sound of exhalation is "hum," which comes from the back of the throat. Try it again. (Brief pause.)

If you are breathing deeply enough, it should become easier to hear. Keep your eyes so that you can better concentrate. Inhale and exhale deeply and listen to your "so hum." Try it a few more times. (Brief pause.)

Every time we breathe, "so hum" comes forth. So hum means "I am He." Your breath reminds you that your identity is connected with the Supreme Soul. You might call it the force, the universal energy, or God. It does not matter what we call it, as long as we understand that we are connected with every breath we take, approximately 15 times a minute, 22 to 23 thousand times a day. The next time that you feel alone or fearful, close your eyes, inhale, exhale, and listen for your reassurance.

Lie down, centered by following your exhalation down, along the imaginary line. Let go until you feel totally released and relaxed—your body loose and limp. Your feet are shoulder width apart and your arms are away from the sides of your body, palms facing up. Relax your facial muscles. Don't squint or frown. Think of something pleasant, smile, and relax your jaw. Take that first breath and listen to your existence, listen to the so hum, the "I am He," of you. You are safe, assured, protected, and loved. Each time you inhale, feel yourself absorbing the universe. Let "It" absorb you. Learn to feel as one with everything—at peace. (Pause a few minutes.)

If an outside thought distracts you, drown it out with your so hum by breathing more deeply, until the disturbance goes away, and return to your restful breathing. (Pause a few minutes.)

Listen to the loud, clear so hum, and hold it with you as you begin to bring your mind and body back to the awareness of the room. Gently stretch your toes, your legs, your arms. Then stretch fully and yawn. Lastly, do whatever your body feels like doing, silently reminding yourself: "My body is relaxed and my mind is peaceful." Smile and join in the celebration of life.

We have been given a gift—a precious gift—LIFE!
If we don't join in the celebration of life by celebrating the Self,
we have no right to that gift.
Pay your debt and honor your Self!
Shanti—Shanti—Shanti—Peace—Peace—Peace

BEGINNER LEVEL LESSON 5

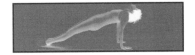

After your first four weeks of yoga, you should begin to feel a little different, more supple in your movements, deeper in your breathing, and calmer in your mind. Yoga is a science of health. Complete health is more than physical. It is mental and spiritual as well. All that you are, or hope to be, depends entirely on you. Your body needs to be stretched and used; your breathing needs to be deep, full, complete. Your mind needs to rest, and your spirit needs inspiration. Body—mind—spirit are all connected and reach their peak in the fulfillment of yoga. This is why you never see an "and" between the words "body" and "mind;" in yoga, it's always "body/mind," "mind/body." No movement, no sitting, no breathing is ever lost or wasted. Each thing we do brings us closer to our goal, closer to health, happiness, and peace.

Alternate Breathing

Breathing through your left or right nostril is called alternate breathing. It helps to cool you down or warm up and is very relaxing. When we are tired, we revive our body by taking a cold or hot shower. We can do the same thing mentally, using our nostrils. Close your right nostril and breathe in through your left. Close the left nostril and breathe out through the right—in through the right and out through the left. Alternate back and forth; it's very calming to the nerves.

Five Ways to Stay Warm: These breathing techniques will help you stay warm on a cold day.

1. Breath out of your right nostril.

2. Sit on the floor with your legs crossed yogi-style, and put your hands on the bottom of your feet. Breathe deeply. You'll begin to feel the warmth circulating throughout your body.

3. Breathe very deeply and slowly. This breathing will keep your circulation moving and create energy and warmth.

4. Sit in a kneeling position on your heels. Lock your hands in front of you and push your elbows side to side very vigorously.

5. Visualize a ball of fire in your stomach as you breathe deeply.

Four Ways to Stay Cool: These breathing techniques will help you stay cool on a hot day.

1. Breathe through your left nostril, closing off the right one.

2. *Sita-kari:* Cooling breath. Open your lips and put your teeth together. Hold your tongue so the tip is behind your lower teeth, and let the air come in sharply as a cooling breath. Close your lips and breathe out through your nose.

3. *Sit-a-li:* Place your tongue between your lips, as though you're holding a straw in your mouth, and suck in the air. Withdraw your tongue, close your lips, and breathe out. Repeat ten times. This action also clears out your sinuses.

4. Mentally cool off. Close your eyes. Breathe deeply and think of snow.

We all want *Satchitananda. Sat* means "existence," *chit* means "knowledge," and *ananda* means "bliss." Yoga is the doorway to existence, knowledge, and bliss. Peace begins through meditation, when you become master of your breath.

 ## Postures to Review

Take the time to just sit and breathe. Pause during the day and check yourself out: How are you breathing? Are you in control? If you find your breath to be short and erratic, you're not in control. Learn to breathe deeply. The deeper you breathe, the more alive you are.

Review all postures from Beginners Lesson 1 (pp. 8–12), performing them in the order given, before trying the new postures.

New Postures

36. Sitting Backward Stretch.

Sit cross-legged on the floor. Inhale and place your hands on the floor behind you. Tilt your pelvis up and let your knees rest on the floor in front of you. Tip your head back. Hold this position as long as you feel it is comfortable. This good stretch relieves the muscles in your thighs and strengthens your shoulders. Exhale when you are ready to come down.

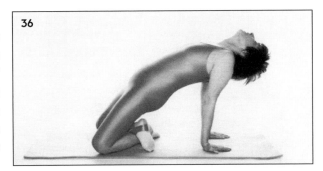

37. Airplane.

This pose is a side stretch or a triangle posture. Stand with your feet comfortably apart. Inhale and raise both arms out straight to the sides, horizontal to the floor. Exhale and bend sideways to your right. Stretch your right arm down your right side as far as you can go, and raise your left arm up in the air. Really stretch your whole left side. Inhale and raise your body back to the starting position. Repeat for your other side. Bend sideways to your left and stretch your left arm down, while lifting your right arm in the air. Exhale and relax your arms down to your sides. Try to keep your arms and knees straight. During this posture, make sure you do not bend forward—keep your movement sideways. To check if you are bending forward, stand with your heels and back against a wall. Raise both arms and bend sideways. Your shoulders, buttocks, and heels should remain touching the wall.

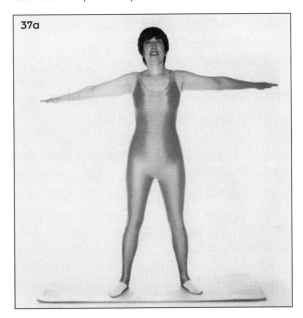

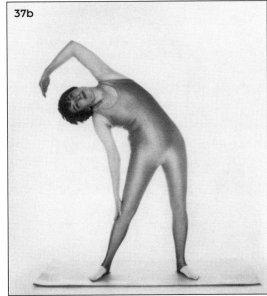

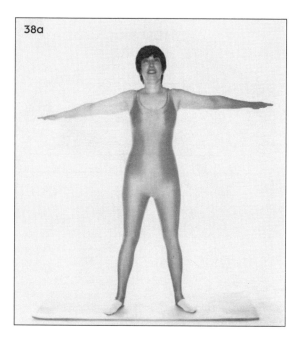

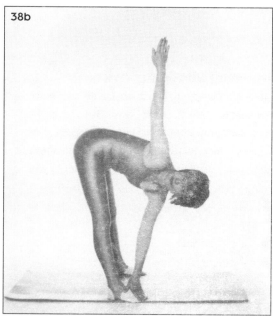

38. Standing Twist.

Stand with your legs as far apart as you can without feeling discomfort. Inhale and raise your arms out to the sides. Raise your left arm up in the air and twist to the left. Exhale and bring your right hand down to your left foot. Turn your head, and look up at your left hand in the air. This movement creates a twist in the spine and the waist. Inhale and lift your body up, bringing your right arm up to a horizontal position again. Repeat for the other side. Raise your right arm up in the air and twist to the right Exhale and bring your left hand down to your right foot, keeping your eyes on the right arm in the air. Inhale and bring your left arm up. Exhale and slowly lower both arms to your sides.

39. Anterior Stretch.

Sit on the floor with your legs stretched out in front of you. As you inhale, lean back and place your hands on the floor behind you. Lift the pelvic area up so you look like a slant board. Look up at the ceiling. Try to keep your arms straight. Hold for a few moments. Exhale and gently lower your body back to a sitting position.

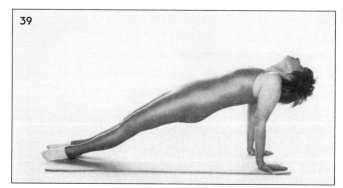

40. Plow and Variations.

First Variation: Lie on your back on the floor with your arms at your sides. Inhale and lift both legs straight up. Keeping your legs straight, lift your buttocks and lower your legs toward your body, over your head, as far as you can without straining. Try to place your toes on the floor behind you. Hold for a few moments. You may support your lower back with your hands. Inhale to come out of the posture. Lift your legs up, keeping them straight, and slowly lower your buttocks and legs to the floor.

Second Variation: Lie on your back with your arms stretched back on the floor behind your head. Let your palms face the ceiling. Inhale. Lift your buttocks, raise your legs like in the first variation, and place your toes on your fingertips. Try to keep your legs straight.

Third Variation: Lie on the floor. Stretch your arms back behind your head and rest them on the floor, palms facing the ceiling. Inhale and lift your buttocks. Raise your legs as in the first variation and bend your knees toward your shoulders.

Fourth Variation: Lie on your back on the floor, keeping your arms by your sides. As you inhale, lift your buttocks and raise your legs as you did in the first variation. Bring your hands up to support your lower back. As you exhale, bend your knees and lower both knees onto your right shoulder Rest in this position for as long as you are comfortable. Inhale and raise your knees to the center. Exhale and lower them to your left shoulder. Inhale to come back to the center, and raise your legs straight into the air. Exhale and slowly and gently lower your body back to the floor. This movement allows you to change position while in an inverted posture.

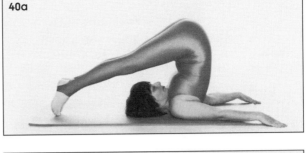

40a

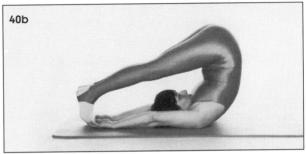

40b

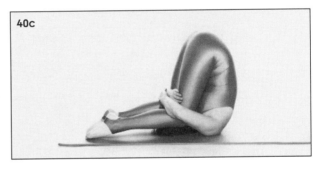

40c

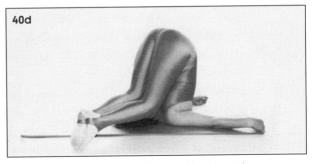

40d

The Plow is a very important posture, particularly for women. Practiced every day, it can alleviate a number of female discomforts. In addition to being a slimming posture, the Plow relieves a multitude of problems: headaches, hangovers, sinus congestion, sciatica, sexual debility, hemorrhoids, constipation, depression, and indigestion. It helps in the regulation of diabetes because of its benefit to the pancreas. Rolling out of this posture by slowly rounding your back is very good for separating the vertebrae and stretching your spine. Inverted positions also give our organs a chance to rest and relax from their usual vertical position.

41. Pelvic Lift.

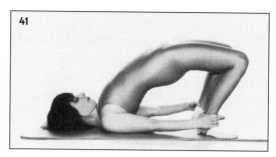

This posture should be done following any of the Plow variations. After the body has been inverted, it should be lifted. Lie on your back, flat on the floor. Raise your knees and bring your heels as close to your buttocks as you can. Hold on to your heels with your hands. Inhale and lift your pelvic area up off the floor as high as you can. Keep your feet flat on the floor. Hold the posture for as long as you are comfortable. Exhale and gently lower your body down. Release your heels and stretch out your legs. Take a nice, deep relaxing breath. For women, the Pelvic Life alleviates menstrual discomfort and is a good toning exercise for before and after childbirth.

42. Three-Quarter Shoulder Stand.

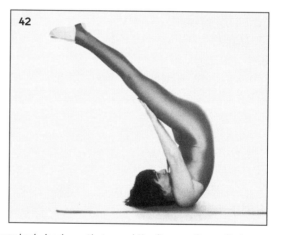

This pose is also called Pose of Tranquillity. Lie on your back with your arms at your sides. Inhale and lift your legs straight up in the air. Raise your arms straight up toward the ceiling with your palms facing your legs. Lift your buttocks and your lower body off the floor, letting your legs fall slightly so that your kneecaps rest in the palms of your hands. Keep your knees straight. Your arms should not be holding you. You should be balancing yourself on your shoulders. Be careful that you do not strain your neck by using it to maintain your balance. If you feel unsteady, roll your body back gently toward the floor until you find your balancing point again. When you are ready to come out of the posture, gently drop your buttocks to the floor, and slowly lower your arms and legs. Take a deep relaxing breath. It takes much practice to perform this posture correctly and to find the balance point that is right for your body. Once you find that point, you will understand why this posture is called the Pose of Tranquillity.

The Shoulder Stand's toning action on the nervous system and circulation helps reduce excess fat. It is also one of the most beneficial postures, relieving depression, regulating diabetes (not a cure), emphysema, sciatica, asthma, bronchitis, colds, sinus problems, indigestion, insomnia, hemorrhoids, neurasthenia, rheumatism, sexual debility, varicose veins, and wrinkles.

Relaxation/Meditation: Complete Relaxation II

Begin by stretching out in the centered, reclining position. Remind yourself that this is your time to let go. Take a very deep inhalation and let out a complete exhalation. Become loose and limp. This is your time to forget about the demands of the clock, the hurry of the day, and to just pause. Remember how a dog flops on the floor, totally and naturally relaxed. Exhalation allows our bodies to go limp. Every time you exhale, to say "limp" to yourself.

Begin by inhaling and raising your left leg a few inches off the floor. Shake it gently. As you exhale, let it fall or collapse to the floor. Do the same thing with your right leg. Inhale and lift your right leg a few inches off the floor. Shake it gently. Exhale and let it fall to the floor.

Inhale and bend your left arm. Rest your elbow on the floor and gently shake your hand, wrist, and fingers. Exhale and let it flop to the floor. Do the same with your right arm. Leave your elbow resting on the floor. Inhale and raise your arm. Gently shake your hand, wrist, and fingers. Exhale and let it fall to the floor.

Inhale and raise your entire left arm a few inches off the floor and shake it gently. On your exhale, let it fall limply back to the floor. Repeat this movement with your right arm. Inhale and lift it a few inches off the floor. Shake your arm gently. Exhale and let it go limp to the floor.

With as little effort as possible, inhale and lift your buttocks off the floor. Exhale and let yourself fall limp to the floor.

On your inhalation, lift your chest and upper abdomen off the floor, arching your back slightly. Exhale and return to the floor.

Starting at your toes and moving to the top of your head, visualize each part of your body going loose and limp—released and relaxed. Go slowly. Do not miss any part of your body. (Pause.)

Your mind is in charge. Tell it to be firm as it orders each part of your body to relax. Remember that a complete exhalation is your best helper in accomplishing this goal. (Pause again.)

Don't forget your head and your neck. Gently roll your head from side to side to relax the neck area, until you are comfortable, and rest there.

We often forget about the tension we hold in our face. Think about relaxing your eyes. Open and close your eyelids very slowly a few times. Let them grow heavier and heavier each time, until you simply let them rest closed, as though you're dozing off to sleep. Finally, relax your jaw by smiling. (Brief pause.)

Twenty minutes of yoga correct relaxation has the restorative powers of two hours of sleep. Sleep is not always relaxing, often filled with disturbing dreams. In yoga, we have no dreams for we let our breath empty our minds. (Pause a few minutes.)

When you are ready to return to your wakeful state, stretch your feet, your legs, your arms, your entire body. Give yourself a positive thought: "My body is relaxed and my mind is peaceful." Stretch fully, twist, turn, yawn, and take a deep inhalation of energy as you rise. Don't forget to smile. It tells the world that you are in charge but, more importantly, it tells *you* that you are in charge.

Listen, really LISTEN to your body.
It talks to you continually. Hear the gentle whispers.
When it shouts, it's probably too late.

What does it want? What does it need?
To be stretched? To relax? To cry or laugh?
Is it hungry? Calm? Agitated?
It needs your attention.
It can only serve you to the extent that you heed its warnings, its pleadings,
its requirements.
Shhhhhhhh—LISTEN!
Shanti—Shanti—Shanti—Peace—Peace—Peace

BEGINNER LEVEL LESSON 6

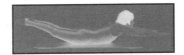

Most of us come to yoga for three reasons. We want to take care of our body. We want to learn to relax, to calm down. We may also feel that our life is not complete. We're searching for some form of happiness, but don't know how to obtain it. In order to be happy, we must find a sense of true peace. The way to true peace is through relaxation and letting go. We can only discover who and what we really are by learning to unwind our body and slow, and finally stopping, our mind with proper breathing.

The Eightfold Path of Yoga

In following this path, we achieve the blissful state found in meditation. Enlightenment and union can result only within the dimensions and to the depths of the individual's ethics and code of conduct. The more you practice within this path, the more successful you will be in finding your state of bliss or permanent joy. The first two aspects of the eightfold path of yoga are yama and niyama, which cover our code of ethics and conduct.

Yama: The Five Restraints

In order to follow the eightfold path of yoga, we practice yama, or the "five restraints." These are:

1. Inoffensiveness. This asks that we not abuse any living things. We should be gentle toward all things. There should be no destruction, no injury, no killing, no abuse of any living thing. We should feel gentleness toward all things and have no destructive impulses or thoughts.

2. Truthfulness. We should not lie, present half-truths, or be evasive. We should refrain from embellishing the facts and should describe things as they really are. Truthfulness does not hurt others. A Hindu proverb tells us: "Speak the truth, speak the pleasant, but not the unpleasant truth." A joke follows this proverb: There was a Hindu doctor whose job was to bring babies into the world. Each time the doctor gave the newborn baby to the mother, the mother would say: "Oh, doctor, isn't my baby the most beau-

tiful baby in the whole world?" Even though the doctor loved babies very much, sometimes the baby wasn't as beautiful as other babies. However, the doctor did not want to lie, so he would respond by saying: "Now *that's* a baby!" This reaction made the new mother feel happy, and the doctor didn't lie. In other words, we should always consider the effects of what we say.

3. Not stealing. In addition to not stealing from another's property, we should also abstain from greediness of any sort. If we are accumulating material things that we really don't need, we're wasting goods, stealing from humankind, and being cruel. Instead of taking, we should wait until offered. We will then become more patient and reflective.

4. Nondesire. Wanting things that belong to others shows a certain amount of jealousy within us. Jealousy generally creates animosity toward the person who possesses what we desire. Our jealousy might lead us to do unwise things, such as steal or go into debt.

5. Continence. It is important to practice self-control and moderation in food and sex. We should eat to live, not live to eat. Our body is sacred and we should do our best to keep it in good shape. Overeating makes us sluggish and interferes with our meditation by making us want to sleep instead. We should enjoy, not abuse, all our senses, even appetite. We don't necessarily have to give up sex, but we should avoid excessive indulgence.

Niyama: The Five Observances

Hand in hand with yama is the practice of *niyama*, or the "five observances," practices that yogis and yoginis follow in order to reach enlightenment. These are:

1. Purification. We must strive to cleanse our body, our mind, and our heart. We must cleanse our mind and heart of hatred, envy, jealousy, anger, greed, lust, and impure thoughts and words. Our body should be kept clean not only by scrubbing it, but also by eating healthy food and keeping it free of pain.

2. Contentment. We should make an honest effort to accept, without resentment or bitterness, all that comes our way, even though it may be disagreeable to us at times.

3. Strength of Character. We should be patient, disciplined, accepting, calm, and follow the five restraints of yama.

4. Study. We should try to read good books, preferably scriptures or anything that is beneficial for our growth.

5. Complete self-surrender to a Higher Being. Wow! This appears to be asking a lot of us. By surrendering the "self," you are giving up your ego-self. In doing so, you will recognize why, who, and what you are. You'll be able to use this knowledge to help others. You will have a genuine desire to experience the present and to know the NOW.

Postures to Review

Breathe. Rest and relax your body. Release all stress, tension, and problems of the day. Then, begin your postures.

Review all postures from Beginners Lesson 1 (pp. 8–12), performing them in the order given, before trying the new postures.

New Postures

43. Upper and Lower Rolls.

Upper Roll: Lie on your back on the floor, and bring your knees to your chest. Your arms are on the floor at your sides. Rock backward and forward from your shoulders to your waist, only using your upper back. Do not let your buttocks touch the floor. Your hands on the floor are used for support. Just roll on your upper back a few times. Lower your legs to the floor.

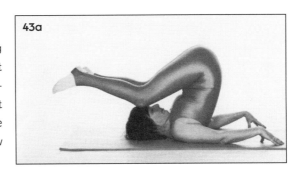

Lower Roll: Lie on your back on the floor. Raise your knees toward your body and cross your legs. Hold your ankles with your hands and roll your waist and hip area around the floor—left to right and right to left. Try to make a big circle, from your waist, to your right side, to your lower back and left side. This movement really makes the lumbar area feel relaxed, and massages the lower back muscles.

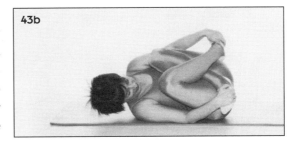

44. Half and Full Bow.

Note: the Bow positions should not be performed if you are suffering from peptic ulcer, hernia, or thyroid or endocrine gland disorders.

Half Bow: Lie on your stomach with your legs apart and your arms stretched out beyond your head. Inhale and lift your arms and legs off the floor, balancing yourself on your stomach. Exhale and slowly lower your arms and legs.

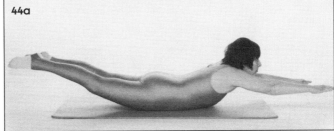

Full Bow: Lie on your stomach and bend your knees up. Stretch your arms back and clasp your hands around your ankles. Inhale and lift your body up, balancing yourself on your stomach. Exhale and lower your body. Unclasp your ankles and lower your legs and arms. Rest.

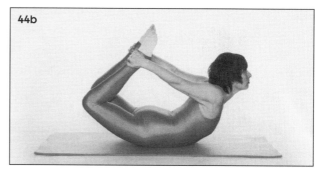

The Bow posture massages abdominal muscles and organs, and thus helps relieve gastrointestinal disorders, constipation, upset stomach, and a sluggish liver. It reduces abdominal fat and aids in rectifying a hunched back.

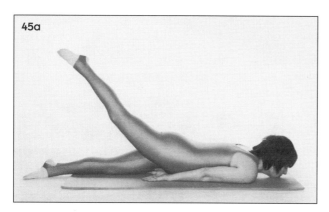

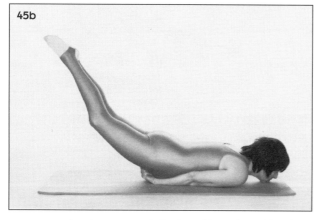

45. Half and Full Locust.

Half Locust: Lie on your stomach with your arms at your sides. Turn your arms inward so that the palms of your hands are under your thighs. Inhale and lift one leg up as high as you can—aim for the ceiling—and hold for as long as you find this position comfortable. Exhale and lower your leg slowly. Repeat for your other leg.

Full Locust: Lie on your stomach with your arms at your sides. Instead of placing your hands under your thighs, as in Half Locust, make your hands into fists. Try to rest your body on the full length of your arms. Push both fists into the floor. Inhale and lift both legs up at the same time, again aiming for the ceiling. Exhale and slowly lower your legs down. This is an important posture that uses almost every muscle in your body. Lie still for a moment and rest.

The Locust postures alleviate moderate abdominal problems and lower back pain or stiffness, but should not be performed if you have a hernia or an acute back problem. The Half and Full Locust help to relieve insomnia, bronchitis, emphysema, and indigestion, as well as normalize body weight and prevent obesity.

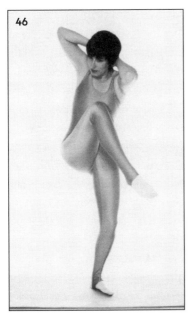

46. Knee to Elbow Lift.

Stand with your hands clasped behind your head. Inhale and lift your right knee up. Bend forward and touch your right knee with your left elbow. Try not to bend downward. The idea is to lift your knee as high as you can. Exhale and lower your knee down, and straighten your body up. Inhale and repeat with your left knee to your right elbow. Follow this movement very slowly, three to four times on each side. Exhale and relax. This posture teaches coordination and balance.

47. Bear Walk and Lower.

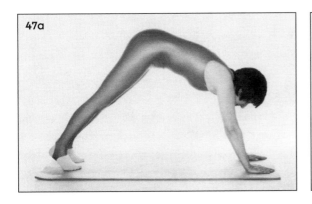 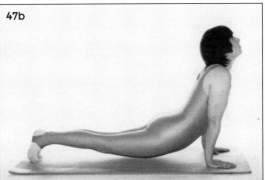

In a standing position, exhale and slowly bend forward and down to the floor. Walk out on your hands, keeping your feet in place, as far as you can comfortably. Lower your body toward the floor. Support yourself with your feet and hands. Look up at the ceiling. This pose is called Lowering the Bear. Raise your body up and walk your hands back to your feet. Pause for a moment. Inhale and lift your body back to a standing position. Exhale.

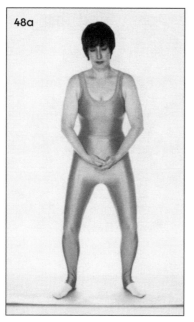

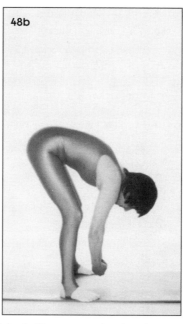

48. Watermelon.

This is a relaxing posture. Stand comfortably with your feet directly below your hips and your hands folded in front of you as if you are holding a very heavy watermelon. Don't think about bending forward. Instead, try to experience the weight of the watermelon. Very slowly, relax your knees and lower your upper body down to the floor.

Relax your knees a little more and open your hands to release the watermelon onto the floor. This posture teaches you to relax and release—relax and let go. Rest in this folded position for a moment.

Relax your knees back and forth. If you are truly relaxed, you may notice your upper body beginning to swing. Inhale and lift your body straight up. Bring your arms over your head. Reach and push up with your arms. Let your arms flow out to your sides as you exhale and bring them back to your waist. Inhale and straighten your knees, while pushing your hands and arms out to the sides. Exhale. Relax your knees and bring your arms back to your waist and down to your sides. Relax.

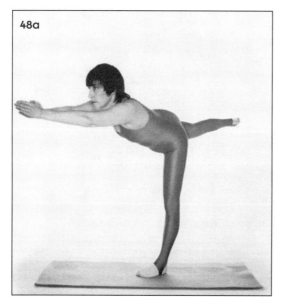

49. Skater.

In a standing position, raise your arms in front of you and place your palms together with your thumbs touching—focus on your thumbs. Inhale and lift one leg up and extend it out behind you. As you extend your leg up and out, bend your body forward, keeping your arms stretched out in front of you and your concentration on your thumbs. Exhale and return to a standing position. Inhale and repeat for your other leg. Exhale and return to a standing position. Rest. This posture is very calming and teaches balance.

Relaxation/Meditation: Cloud Trip

One of the best ways to relax is to become part of nature—to blend into it. This concept may sound a bit strange if you have never tried it, but with practice, you will gain a better understanding of the pleasure found in nature.

Begin by relaxing your body comfortably, centered to the floor. Settle in by twisting, turning, or wiggling a little. Remember to exhale deeply and thoroughly to release the tightness you've accumulated during your daily life movements. Release yourself to peace and tranquillity. When your body is comfortable, prepare to go on a cloud trip.

Instead of lying in your present room, picture yourself stretched out on a small hill, resting on a soft plot of grass. Sink into the grass and let go. It feels warm and comfortable, and you feel relaxed, safe, secure, and serene. You desire nothing. You feel complete, content, calm, cozy. Above you stretches a pale blue sky that makes you feel even more peaceful. Feel the sun on your face and the cool breeze passing over you. You are free of all anxieties, all worries and wants. And look, there's a bird doing loop-de-loops and swirls in the sky—flying free. Yet lying there, you come to realize that freedom is not so much in the movement of flight, but in your present stillness of mind.

A soft, billowy, white cloud comes into view. You watch it drift along, until you realize it has paused right above you. Listen to what it is saying to you. It's inviting you to come aboard. Don't hesitate. Don't be afraid to climb aboard. You'll be safe. Stretch out and sink in. It feels like a feather bed.

Trust. Relax and let go. Just drift around and experience what feeling carefree is all about, as a puff of wind lifts you upward. You feel unhampered, unrestricted, free. Effortlessly, you drift along, riding the breeze, totally relaxed in the moment. Indeed, you have never felt so free, so unburdened and at rest. It's as if you were the cloud, with all its attributes. Where do you begin and where does the cloud end? The answer is not important. Allow yourself to drift awhile. Feel the lightness, the freedom, and the peace. (Pause for a few minutes.)

Hold on to this sense of peace as your cloud drifts back over the grass. As your cloud pauses, you climb down, back to your spot on the grass, and watch as it slowly drifts from your sight, further and further away, getting smaller and smaller until it's gone. It is gone, but not the feeling of being on that cloud. You still feel rested and renewed, revived. All pressures and pains have left you. All anger and anxiety, fear and frustration are gone. You feel empty but full, complete and at one with yourself. Fill yourself with this quiet joy. And know that perfect peace is always deep inside you, waiting to come out. When you take the time to pause, to be quiet and still, to absorb and to be absorbed, then you will experience this oneness that is lovingness. The word "joy" will have a new meaning for you. (Brief pause.)

When you return to your surroundings, bring your experience with you. Hold on to it as you gently stretch yourself back to aliveness. Fully stretch and yawn. Follow whatever your body needs to do at this moment, while still holding on to your positive thought: "My body is relaxed and my mind is peaceful." Smile.

The sun smiles to you. Smile back.
The star winks to you. Wink back.
The winds caress you. The waters refresh you. The trees send you oxygen.
The cricket chirps you to sleep. The songbird awakens you.
How can you step outdoors and not feel grateful and not say "Thank you!"
Shanti—Shanti—Shanti—Peace—Peace—Peace

BEGINNER LEVEL LESSON 7

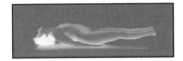

The third step of the eightfold path of yoga is the asanas—the postures. We could do all eight hundred and forty thousand of them, but that would take a little time; probably more time than most of you want to dedicate to it. When most people think of yoga the first, and sometimes only, thought that comes to their mind is "postures." While the postures are vitally important they are only a part of yoga. There has to be much more to yoga for it to be called "our second chance at life."

Asanas: The Postures

Yoga is concerned with both the outer and inner movements of the body. The internal and external go hand in hand, just as proper breathing and the execution of postures go hand in hand. Every posture in yoga is beneficial in some way to some part of our body. It can range from something as simple as extending your tongue, which prevents sore throats, to standing on your head, which supplies fresh blood to vital cells, can prevent senility, and benefits the pituitary gland. Practicing as few as ten postures a day, along with a healthy diet, can keep your body in good shape. Yoga is not a miracle. It is common sense, which we sometimes forget to use.

Always be sure that you do some form of twist posture each day to keep your spine supple, flexible, alive! Do an inverted posture to give your organs a rest from the down-pull that is a result of our constant vertical position in life. Be sure to do a balance position each day. They are most calming to the nerves. Remember the yoga saying: "Old age begins in the joints; you'll be stiff long enough without allowing it to happen while you're still alive." We move in a practiced, ramrod style of walking all day long, holding back or being uptight. Learn to give both your body and mind a break by moving more spontaneously, more freely, more lightly at certain times during each day. Yoga will help you to stay flexible enough to achieve this goal. Yoga can assist you to recapture the freedom of movement of your youth. Is yoga the fountain of youth? No, it is the fountain of life!

Pranayama: Breath

Step four on the eightfold path of yoga is *pranayama*—breathing. Breathing is a physical means to a spiritual end. Regulated breathing helps control your mind. Your breath is an energy that you draw from the universe that surrounds you. It is a life force. As you inhale, think of the pure prana energy, the life-giving force entering your body. Hold it and think your mantra, a spiritual thought or life force. Some think of the word "Om"—God. As you exhale, think about the impurities leaving your body.

Every thought affects you. You are what you think. There is no greater truth. What you think during your breathing affects your whole being. Controlled breath determines everything in your life. It is the road that leads to success in meditation. It is your life.

Pratyahra: Nerve Control

Number five on the eightfold path of yoga is *pratyahara*—the complete withdrawal of the senses and the relaxation of every organ. Literally, pratyahara means "nerve control." It is emptying your mind in order to be able to concentrate. It is only through proper concentration that you can learn to meditate. The average mind has four thousand thoughts a minute. Pratyahara helps us control our scattered thoughts by helping our mind become very still. When you sit quietly, let your mind wander from thought to thought, subject to subject, like a grasshopper jumping all around. Allow yourself to observe your mind, but don't try to control it. The next time you decide to sit quietly again, you'll notice that your mind is less turbulent, more calm. When you continue this practice over a period of weeks, months, or even years you'll learn to be able, at will, to free your mind from your brain. The mind is sometimes like a child who wants to get your attention. If you ignore the child, it will settle down. Let your mind settle down, and let it become still.

 ## Postures to Review

Breathe deeply and release all stress. Release and relax your body before you begin your postures.

Review all postures from Beginners Lesson 1 (pp. 8–12), performing them in the order given, before trying the new postures.

New Postures

50. Standing Backward Stretch.

Standing with your feet comfortably apart and your arms at your sides, inhale and lift your arms over your head. Stretch as though your whole body is reaching for the ceiling. Really stretch your spine. Lean back slightly. Exhale. Let your arms fall out to your sides and gently come back to an upright position.

51. Standing Waist Roll.

Stand comfortably with your hands on your hips. Roll your waist and bend your body forward to the left side, to the back, to the right side, and back to the front. Do these rolls three or four times. Begin your rotation to the left, then reverse and rotate to the right. This pose loosens up your waist and slims it down; it also loosens the spine.

52. Windmill.

Stand comfortably. Lift your arms out to your sides and swing them vigorously, making circles backward. Slowly, come to a stop and reverse the motion. Swing vigorously making forward circles. Exhale and let your arms relax to your sides. This is an energizing posture. If you stand with your eyes closed, you will become aware of all the energy inside you, and you will feel very alive.

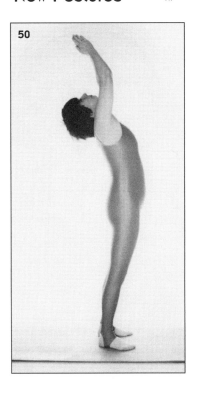

53. Rowing.

Sit on the floor with your legs straight out in front of you. Raise your arms parallel to your legs. Stretch forward, all the way to your toes, as though you were holding on to a pair of oars. Lean backward as far as you can, almost lying flat on the floor, and pull the oars back to your chest. Reach forward with your oars and pull back. Inhale as you bring the oars to your chest, and exhale as you stretch forward. Repeat this movement very slowly, six to eight times. This posture teaches us to sit up and is also good for the stomach muscles.

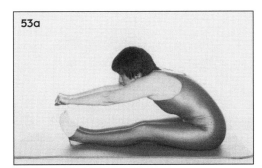

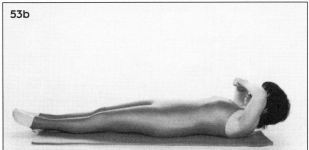

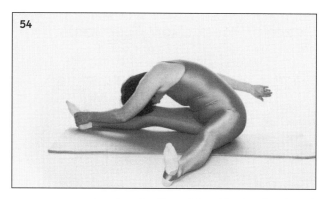

54. Sitting Twist Swing.

Sit on the floor and open your legs to your comfort level. Inhale and lift your arms out to your sides. Exhale and twist from the waist to your right. Stretch forward and place your left hand on your right toe. As you twist at the waist, reaching for your toe, your right arm swings behind you as far as possible. Inhale and return to center. Exhale. Twist, stretch your right hand to your left toe, and swing your left arm behind you. This is a good posture for the waist and for keeping the spine loose. It should be practiced four to five times on each side.

55. Sitting Mill.

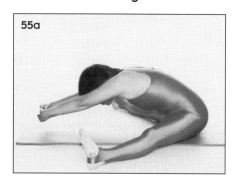
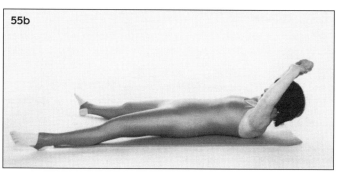

Sit on the floor with your legs comfortably apart. Interlace your fingers and face the palms of your hands outward. Stretch forward and push your arms out in front of you. You are going to be making a large circle. Stretch and rotate to the right. Lean back and pull your arms to your chest. Stretch and rotate to the left, stretching your arms out. Rotate back to the center. Stretch and push as far as you can. Reverse your rotation, and repeat this movement three to four times each way. This posture loosens the spine.

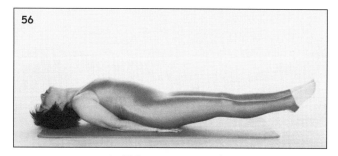

56. Advanced Fish Lift.

Go into the Fish posture (number 5, on p. 9). Lie on your back on the floor. Slightly raise your upper body, keeping the top of your head on the floor and your arms stretched out on your thighs. From your Fish position, lift both legs three or four inches off the floor. Keep your legs straight and hold the pose for a few moments. This posture strengthens your stomach and thigh muscles.

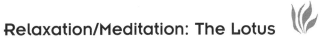

Relaxation/Meditation: The Lotus

Stretch out and center your body comfortably on the floor. Keep your legs about 18 inches apart and your arms away from your sides with your palms facing upward. Adjust your head comfortably—your neck, face, and jaw relaxed. Follow your exhalation to help you in your relaxation. With each exhalation, allow yourself to sink deeper and deeper into peacefulness.

With your eyes closed, visualize a beautiful pond. At the center of this very still pond rest, a very large, white lotus flower. Behold this flower for a moment with all its serenity.

Imagine that you can see right down to the center of that lotus flower. At the very center of the flower is a small dark spot. Keep looking at that spot in the center of the flower. It grows larger as you watch it. Keep watching as it gets bigger and bigger. Something wonderful will happen very soon. Watch. (Brief pause.)

A little figure is sitting right in the center of the lotus flower. Keep looking at that figure for it too will soon begin to grow larger and larger. (Brief pause.)

You realize that this figure is *you*. Watch yourself lean back, stretch out, and sink right into the center of this gigantic flower. Your face is lifted to a soft, warm, caressing sun. Enjoy the breeze, and breathe as gently as the breeze. Feel free and blissful. (Brief pause.)

Experience your body's release of tightness and tension. Is your mind calm and content? Is your breath effortlessly flowing? Fill yourself with this moment of bliss. (Brief pause.)

The sun has gently blanketed your body into warmth. As it disappears behind a passing cloud, you feel a gentle warmth from the huge lotus petals that cradle and caress you like a huge hand. You feel protected, safe, and loved. Your only thought is: "At last, I am at peace." (Brief pause.)

The gigantic lotus petals slowly begin to fold outward again, and the you in the center begins to grow smaller and smaller, until you are once again back in your practice room. Your body is back, but your mind is still filled with the peace and love of the lotus. Know that you'll return again.

Slowly awaken your body back to aliveness with a very subtle first stretch, like the first half-awake stretch in the morning. Continue with a full stretch, a twist, a turn, a releasing yawn, and an energizing inhalation. Allow yourself to smile and be grateful for having touched peacefulness once more. Take this final thought: "Life is a celebration."

Shall you pray or meditate? It depends.

If you want to "talk" to God, then, pray.

If you want God to talk to you, meditate.

Which is best?

You will learn more from listening, particularly to the wordless, to the silence.

Judge for yourself, but be honest in your judging.

And, remember, all answers do not come in words.

Shanti—Shanti—Shanti—Peace—Peace—Peace

BEGINNER LEVEL LESSON 8

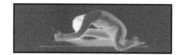

Yogi or yogini—spiritually developed people—find happiness through meditation. Samadhi—enlightenment and bliss—can never truly be described, for how does one put the infinite into finite words? But it can be experienced! Some have called enlightenment touching the center of the cosmos. Others have said that it was like doing a somersault without moving and being in the center of the past, present, and future all at once with no awareness of time. When I briefly enter into deep meditation, I am suddenly filled with a quiet knowing—knowing as I have never known, as if I have spent my entire life looking out through curtains and suddenly the curtains are gone! The utter comfort of that quiet knowing is like nothing else that I have ever experienced. When you open yourself to possibility and allow it to happen, you too can experience this knowing and this new sight. The next three steps in the eightfold path of yoga move further toward an enlightened state of being.

Dharana: Concentration

The sixth stage of the eightfold path of yoga is *dharana*—concentration or mind control. You begin by concentrating on different parts of the body. For example, you might concentrate on your third eye, the area right above your nose. You might choose to concentrate on your heart or your navel. Later in your practice, you can begin to concentrate on an object of your own choice, as long as it is something beautiful or inspiring or something from nature. It must be a pure thought. Concentration is allowing your mind to flow uninterrupted toward the same object for twelve seconds. Although, it might sound simple, it takes much practice to be able to reach dharana.

In concentration, you establish a subject-object relationship with the object you choose to focus on. In meditation, however, you'll find yourself becoming the object and moving beyond all self-imposed limits.

Dhyana: Meditation

Step seven in the eightfold path of yoga is *dhyana*—meditation. Concentration becomes meditation when the chosen object is no longer of a material nature, but of a spiritual nature. It is said in yoga that concentration is the mark of genius, but that meditation is the mark of saintliness. Meditation is a continual flow of energy minus the ego. When you meditate you merge your consciousness with the universal consciousness. Concentration always involves only the mind, and is a function of the ego's concerns, while meditation involves the heart and the whole being.

Samadhi: Pure Consciousness

The first seven steps on the eightfold path of yoga bring us to the final step—*samadhi*—pure consciousness, and the ultimate goal of yoga. Samadhi is spiritual enlightenment, ultimate bliss. Enlightenment is the highest spiritual state you can attain here on earth. Your mind becomes free of any desire of the ego and merely observes and contemplates with nonattachment.

When the last three stages of the eightfold path of yoga—dharana, dhyana, and samadhi—are combined, they are referred to as *samyana*. When you open yourself to possibility and allow it to happen, you too can experience this knowing and this new sight.

Postures to Review

Breathe, relax your body, and leave the cares of the day outside the door. Breathe away all your stress and tension. Breathe into right now. Rest and begin your postures.

Review all postures from Beginners Lesson 1 (pp. 8–12), performing them in the order given, before trying the new postures.

New Postures

57. Lotus Relaxed Posture.

Sit on the floor with your legs out straight in front you. Inhale and bend your left leg and place your left foot next to your buttocks. Exhale and extend your body down over your right leg. Try to put your head to your knee. Inhale and return to a sitting position. Exhale. Inhale and bend your right leg and place your right foot next to your buttocks Extend your left leg out in front of you. Exhale and extend your body down over your left leg. Inhale and return to a sitting posi-

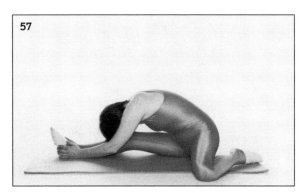

tion. Try to keep the extended leg straight. Remember not to force your body into doing something that is not comfortable.

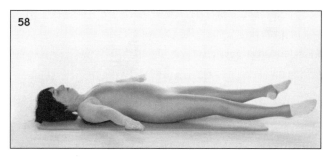

58. Instant Corpse.

Lie on your back on the floor with your legs slightly apart and your arms relaxed at your sides. Inhale and lift your arms and legs three to four inches off the floor. Hold the pose. Exhale and slowly lower yourself down.

The Corpse pose stimulates blood circulation and exercises your vital organs. It alleviates fatigue, neurasthenia, asthma, constipation, diabetes (not a cure), indigestion, insomnia, lumbago, back and neck aches, depression, and sinus problems. It also fosters mental concentration.

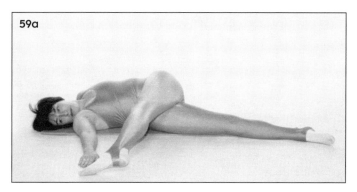

59. Lying Scissors.

First Position: Lie on your back on the floor with your arms out to your sides, your shoulders high, and your palms down. Inhale and lift your left leg straight up. Exhale and cross your left leg over your body. Try to touch your left toes with your right hand. Keep your shoulders flat on the floor. Inhale and lift your left leg up. Exhale and lower it back to the floor. Inhale and lift your right leg up. Exhale and cross your right leg over your body. Try to touch your right toes to your left hand. Inhale and lift your leg up. Exhale and lower it slowly to the floor.

Second Position: After the first position, remain on the floor. Inhale and lift both legs straight up. Exhale and lower both legs to the right side of your body and try to touch your right hand with your right toes. Inhale and raise your legs up. Exhale and slowly lower them to the floor. Inhale and raise both your legs again. Exhale and lower both your legs to your left side and try touching your left hand with your toes. Inhale to raise your legs. Exhale to lower them to the floor. Throughout this movement, try to keep your legs straight and your shoulders on the floor. This posture is a very good workout for your stomach muscles and your outer thigh muscles. Take a slow, deep breath and relax.

60. Hinge.

Kneel on the floor with your body upright and your arms loosely at your sides. Tighten your buttocks and lean back as far as you can. Hold the posture. Straighten up. Repeat three or four times. You will feel the pull in your thigh muscles.

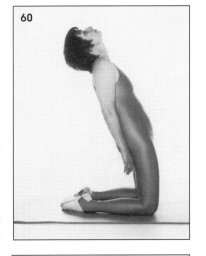

61. Forearm-Wrist Stretch.

Kneel on the floor, but do not sit back on your buttocks yet. Keep your hands on the floor in front of you with your fingers facing forward and your arms straight. Starting with the shoulders, turn your arms outward until your fingers are facing your knees. The palms of your hands should stay flat on the floor. Exhale and gently lean back slightly. You will feel a pull in your wrist area. Inhale and return to center. This is an excellent posture for strengthening the wrists and is particularly helpful for tennis players.

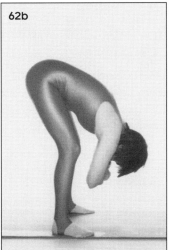

62. Sun Relax.

Stand straight and bring your palms together in front of your body. Overlap your thumbs. Keeping your eyes on your thumbs, raise your arms straight up above your head, and give yourself a gentle stretch. Exhale and keep your arms close to your head. Slowly, lower your arms by letting your elbows come down first. Allow your fingers to come past your face until your arms are at your sides. Relax your chin down to your chest and feel your shoulders relax. Relax your knees, and very slowly relax forward and down to the floor, one vertebra at a time. Let the weight of your body carry you down comfortably. When you have come down as far as you can go, cross your arms over each other and let the weight of your arms hold you down. Take three very slow deep breaths and tell yourself to relax. Let your arms unfold and hang loosely. Inhale to lift your body. Picture each vertebra unfolding gently as your body rises back to a standing position. Exhale. You are relaxed.

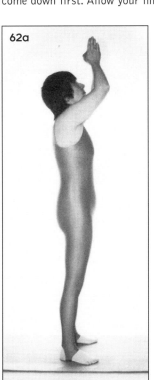

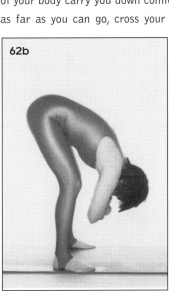

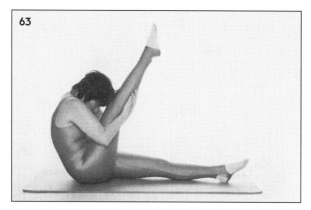

63. Leg Up/Sit Up.

Lie on the floor with your legs out straight and your arms at your sides. Inhale and raise one leg straight up. Raise your torso up to meet your raised leg. Clasp both hands around your knee and touch your head to your knee. Exhale and release your knee, and slowly lower your body and your leg to the floor. Inhale and repeat for the other side. Practice this posture slowly, three to four times for each side, alternating sides.

 ## Relaxation/Meditation: Mind Control

In this session you are going to practice awareness. Begin by sitting fairly straight, and relax without slouching. Close your eyes and take a few relaxing breaths, following your exhalation. (Brief pause.)

Our mind never seems to stop wandering from one thing to another. It is like a child who will do almost anything to get our attention. But as soon as it realizes that we are not paying attention it stops its performance, just as a child will do.

In this session you are just going to let your mind wander wherever it chooses. Do not try to think anything and do not try to control it, simply be aware of the thoughts passing through your mind. You are an observer.

It might help you to picture a large blackboard in front of you. Watch this jumble of thoughts become a group of words running across the blackboard, pass from one side to the other. If you stay detached from these thoughts, they will tire more quickly, and you will be free of them. Try this visualization for a few minutes. (Pause.)

You've just witnessed the congestion that filters through your mind in only a few minutes. Can you see why your mind so desperately needs to rest, to empty out, to be still?

If you find yourself thinking, try to slow down your thoughts and try to make them more enjoyable. To help you learn to control your mind, concentrate on the following phrases. Don't try to analyze them, just concentrate on each one, until you hear the next phrase. You may lie down, but be sure to remain centered and relaxed.

1. "The cat's purr is silent." (Pause.)

2. "The only light is the inner light." (Pause.)

3. "All things are possible when I am with the Absolute." (Pause.)

4. "Let me become what I Am." (Pause.)

5. "Live in the present or the future is a hoax." (Pause.)

6. "I will no longer look—I will see." (Pause.)

7. "Touching a flower, I touch infinity." (Pause.)

8. "Even a pebble disturbs an ocean." (Pause.)

9. "Inside, I find the real 'I Am.' " (Pause.)

10. "I will rest in the 'I Am.'" (Longer pause.)

Learn to recapture the "I Am," and learn to dwell in it. It is your path home, to the peace you seek and the joy you long for. To claim it, you must open yourself to it.

When you are ready to come out of your meditation, gently stretch and pause. As usual, affirm to yourself: "My body is relaxed and my mind is peaceful." Go into your full stretch, your yawn, your deep inhalation of energy. Give in to your body's need to twist or turn. Rise up when you are ready, and smile.

Choose the moment wisely.
For this moment and your decision flow into and affect the next, the next, and the next.
Indeed, you will carry your decision all your life.
Shanti—Shanti—Shanti—Peace—Peace—Peace

BEGINNER LEVEL LESSON 9

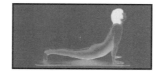

Did you take time to *really* breathe, today? We take time to clean our house of dirt. We rake leaves from our yard and change the air filter in the car, but, all too often, we don't take ten minutes out of our day to just stop and breathe deeply, to clean ourselves physically and mentally. Did you take the time to release tension, anger, frustration, tiredness? Was your mind peaceful? Was your body healthy?

We don't always notice the first signs of tension. Tension can build up over time almost unnoticed, and if left uncared for, it can become fatal. Stress can lead to heart attacks and cancer, and in some cases death. Try conducting a survey of yourself: Are you breathing properly? Don't wait until you want to cry, scream, or run away. Don't wait too long to listen to your body. You must learn to be aware of *you*, because you're the only one who can.

The Five Stumbling Blocks

The following five stumbling blocks are the areas within yourself that should be surveyed and corrected.

1. Disease and pain. An unhealthy person with physical discomforts cannot practice meditation successfully. Even a headache or indigestion interrupts concentration. If we don't exercise or eat healthy food, our body is not healthy, and we are unable to sit still and meditate.

2. Mental laziness. A teacher can only encourage you, but *you* must fight the laziness. Accept each setback as a challenge. There are no failures because each time you sit and breathe and try to meditate, you're that much closer to your goal. Something is always gained.

3. Doubt. This stumbling block is considered the most serious because it can cause your mind to stand still. We must learn to persevere past doubt. Doubt will pass and float away, and a positive state of mind will always return.

4. Lethargy and drowsiness. These stumbling blocks can be attributed to sickness or even overeating. Sometimes it comes from a lack of enthusiasm or from half-heartedness. In any case, it is detrimental to any type of success, from meditation to baking a cake, to making love.

5. Negative emotions. We often dwell too much on the past. Were we clever enough? Did we say something smart enough? We re-live the past, things that hurt our pride, our ego. We also worry about the future. Will we make a good impression? Will we get the job? In doing so, we dwell in the two nonexistent states of time—the past and the future. We forget about the most important time in our lives: *right now. Now* is all we have. We must learn to keep our minds from dwelling on negative emotions, like anger, hate, fear, and panic, which set us back. We must learn to have positive thoughts and step forward. Of course, once in a while, every one of us will get a negative thought, which is acceptable as long as we replace it right away with a positive thought. That's your step forward, for two conflicting thoughts must eventually be settled.

One of the great yogis once said that the most effective antidote to fruitless indulgence and negative emotion is the relaxation of the body combined with slow, deep breathing. As your muscles relax, tension leaves your body and your mind, which gradually becomes calm and once more under control.

Postures to Review

Breathe deeply and relax. Let all stress, all worry, all fears and frustrations leave you.

Review all postures from Beginners Lesson 1 (pp. 8–12), performing them in the order given, before trying the new postures.

New Postures

In the first lesson, you learned fourteen postures; in the next seven lessons, you learned seven new postures each week. This week you will only have one new posture. The Sun Worship/Sun Salutation includes twelve consecutive positions. The entire cycle should be repeated twice in order to work both sides of your body. Begin with your right side (right leg) and repeat on your left side (left leg).

64. Sun Worship/Sun Salutation (see pages 68-69).

Position One: January. Stand with your hands and palms together in front of your chest as in prayer.

Position Two: February. Inhale and reach straight up with your arms over your head. Bend back as far as you comfortably can.

Position Three: March. As you exhale, bend forward and bring your palms to the floor and place them outside your feet. Your legs remain straight.

Position Four: April. Inhale and stretch your right leg back with your left knee bent. Keep your hands in place. Slightly bend your right knee. Arch your back and tip your head to look at the ceiling.

One—January

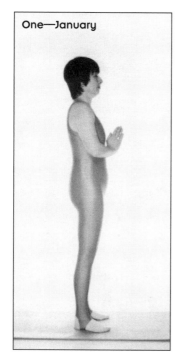

Two—February

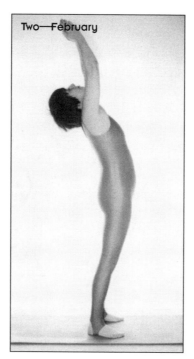

Three—March

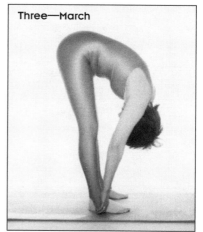

Four—April

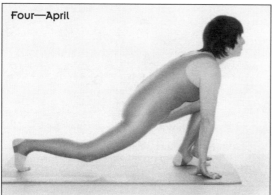

Five—May

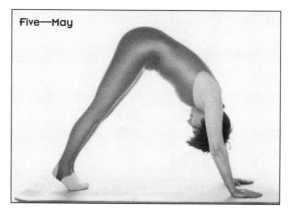

Six—June

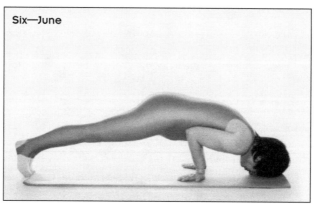

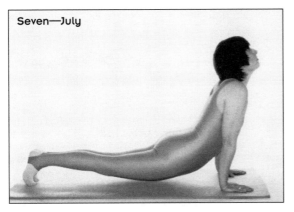

Seven—July

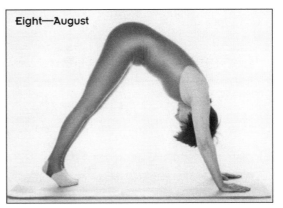

Eight—August

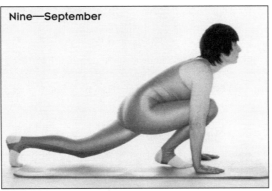

Nine—September

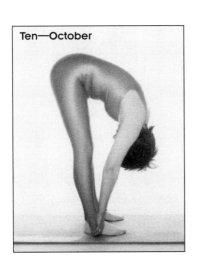

Ten—October

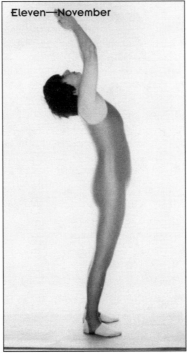

Eleven—November

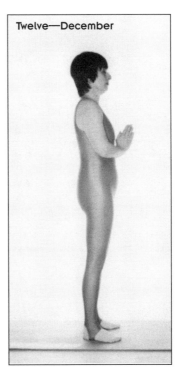

Twelve—December

Position Five: May. Exhale and stretch your left leg back so your feet are parallel and flat on the floor. Get up on your toes and raise your body to make an inverted V. Let your head relax downward.

Position Six: June. Still on your toes, drop down to your knees. Sway back slightly and bring your elbows in to support your rib cage. Bend down to place your nose on the floor. Your hips are slightly raised.

Position Seven: July. Inhale and curve up the front of your body as in Cobra posture.

Position Eight: August. Exhale and raise your hips into the air, making your body into an inverted V and bringing your feet in slightly. Let your head hang down.

Position Nine: September. Inhale and bring your right foot up between your hands. Your left foot should be extended out behind you. Look up at the ceiling.

Position Ten: October. Exhale and bring your left leg up. Place your left foot parallel to your right foot between your hands. You legs should be straight and your body folded together like in position three.

Position Eleven: November. Inhale and raise your body. Stretch your arms up and lean back slightly.

Position Twelve: December. Exhale and bring your palms together in front of your chest. Take a relaxing breath.

Benefits of the Sun Salutation

Positions 1 and 12 establish a state of concentration.

Positions 2 and 11 stretch your abdominal muscles, exercise your arms and spinal cord.

Positions 3 and 10 aid in the prevention and relief of stomach ailments, reduce abdominal fat, improve digestion and circulation, and keep your spine limber.

Positions 4 and 9 tone your abdomen and your thigh and leg muscles.

Positions 5 and 8 strengthen the nerves and muscles of your arms and legs, and exercise your spine.

Positions 6 and 7 strengthen the nerves and muscles of your shoulders, arms, and chest.

 # Relaxation/Meditation: The Third Eye

During the following meditation you will discover your third eye, which is located in the space between, your eyes, one inch up. You may either sit or lie down. If you choose to lie down, be sure to adjust your body in a balanced position.

When you are comfortable and relaxed, imagine that you are looking inside the area between your eyes. It is very, very dark. Concentrate on this darkness and keep looking in at the darkness. (Brief pause.)

Away in the distance, you see a small point of light. It is very far away and very small, but you keep watching it and concentrating on it. You will bring it closer to you. Simply watch as it begins to move closer and closer and grow larger and larger, brighter and brighter, much like the beam of light from a train. (Brief pause.)

It continues to get closer, larger, and brighter. The darkness about the edges has almost disappeared, and there is only this blazing, bright light filling all the darkness that was there. Every corner is filled with light. Notice, however, that, even in its brightness, the light is not glaring or uncomfortable. Its silver glitter gives off a peaceful, warming glow. You can feel it surrounding and covering you, as though you were bathed within it. Pause now in your concentration and enjoy the blanket of warm light that covers you. Feel how it caresses you, like a protective blanket. Notice how it shimmers with its multifaceted beams. It is truly a heavenly light. Rest there a moment. (Pause.)

Hold on to the feeling of being clean and refreshed and bathed in light. Indeed, you are the essence of light. If you can experience this light, you've reached home. If you have not experienced it yet, the time will come when you will.

After having filled yourself with this light, you must let it go back to its source. Still concentrating on the area between your eyes, watch the outer corners begin to turn dark once more, gradually filling in. The width of the light grows narrower and narrower and moves away from you ever so slowly and smoothly. It continues to move away and grow smaller and more distant, until it's gone. It's dark again. Although you see only darkness, you still feel light. The light still covers, warms, and even protects you, and you feel at peace. Simply rest in this peace for a few moments and absorb it as you absorbed the light. Fill yourself with it so that you may take it with you when you leave. (Pause.)

Now that you have looked within and found comfort, you should remember that comfort, peace, and joy can always be found deep within you when you pause long enough to open yourself to this presence. It is about learning to be present in the Presence. When you open yourself, you will blossom, grow, and know.

Think about this blossoming as you bring your body back to aliveness. Like a flower or a plant, that slowly and gently unfolds each petal, unfold yourself into a gentle stretch. Then, as the flower pushes itself up from the soil, push yourself into your full stretch, your twist, your turn, your yawn, your true blossoming. And, just like the flower raises its face to the sun, raise your face and smile.

Listen not as much to the OUTER silence as to the INNER silence.
Listen closely.
Have you realized ALL of you? Or, are you just acquainted with the outer?
Shanti—Shanti—Shanti—Peace—Peace—Peace

BEGINNER LEVEL LESSON 10

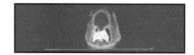

Congratulations! You have completed the first ten-week session; in fact, you should congratulate yourself for finishing something you started—very few people have that much discipline. Success in yoga basically depends on two things: begin and continue. You've done the first so you're halfway there. Don't stop now, go all the way. Continue your search for yourself: from the beginners' lessons that you are now completing, to the intermediates, to the advanced and advance, advance, advance. Never stop!

In this week's lesson, you'll review some of the postures you have learned in these past ten weeks. Take this week to continue solidifying your yoga routine, working on the postures listed below. Next week, you'll go on to the first lesson in the Intermediates level, and spend another week reviewing what you have learned. Hopefully your routine has become a natural part of your day—something you look forward to each morning.

Postures to Review

Perform all postures from Beginners Lesson 1 (pp. 8–12). Next, perform the following postures: Sun Worship; Swan; Floating Swan; Balance on Fours; Cat, Lift, Kick; Infant and Stretch; Forward Frog.

Relaxation/Meditation: Nada-Brahma

Even though yoga is now in the mainstream of alternative health practices, sometimes people are still skeptical and will ask: "You're not going to sit around doing all that mantra chanting, are you?" I can only presume from their question that they either do not really understand the concept of yoga or that they think of yoga as some sort of religious fanaticism. Yoga is not about teaching religion or changing anyone's religious beliefs. Yoga is about bringing body/mind/spirit into perfect harmony. It is about being healthy physically, calm and content mentally, and about touching our inner spiritual nature, our real Self.

In the following meditation, you will not chant a mantra, but you will hum. This meditation is called Nada-Brahma, and is a Tibetan practice. Humming is universal, regardless of your origin, or whether you practice yoga or not. Your mother probably hummed to you when you were a baby, and it soothed you. A cat's purr is a form of humming.

Humming creates a vibration throughout your body. It is relaxing at any pitch. You don't have to worry about breathing properly, and there are no words to remember. Words can be a distraction to relaxation. Humming should be performed effortlessly, almost automatically. Do not force it. If you become tired of humming, simply be silent for a few moments, and rest in the sound.

Close your eyes and go within yourself. Sit and hum for 5 to 10 minutes and allow yourself to experience the vibration you create. (Take a long pause of 5 to 10 minutes to experience the vibration.)

Keep feeling this vibration as you lie back, right where you are, keeping your eyes closed. Adjust your body comfortably on the floor. All sounds of the universe are one gigantic hum. Even in the midst of a large city, with all its different sounds, we can hear a gigantic hum. Humming to ourselves, we join in the chorus of the universe. We experience its vibrations and feel a closeness, a oneness to all things. A magnificent joining takes place, and a togetherness happens. Just as the in-breath and the out-breath are the same breath, the universal hum and your hum are the same. The more we hum, the more we join in and truly experience the universal breath. When you feel this union, there will be no more mysteries to confuse you or questions to ask, only a very quiet, positive knowing. You will have reached the harmony of your existence that you longed for. Learn to hum with the universe—be not only in it, but of it, as indeed you are. Namaste. We are one.

> *Know that you are of a circle and circles never end.*
> *They only encompass and include all that there is.*
> *Just as you are in the world, so all the world is within you.*
> *If you allow and awaken to it.*
> *Rub your eyes. Wake up.*
> *Stretch to your new understanding that you are precious and perfect—just as you are!*
> *Shanti—Shanti—Shanti—Peace—Peace—Peace*

Intermediate Level Lessons

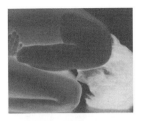

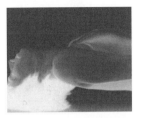

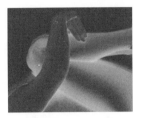

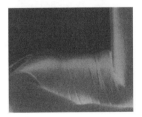

INTERMEDIATE LEVEL LESSON 1

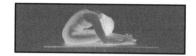

In my classroom, I begin the Intermediates session with a review of the foundation asanas. For you, this is your second week of review, and you might want to move on to new postures. However, it's important that you patiently take your time and become completely familiar with the postures, so you won't have to rely on this book all the time. When you really know your postures, you can go anywhere and stay healthy because your exercise equipment is all in your body/mind! The more comfortable you are with the foundation yoga postures, the better you will be able to perform the intermediate postures. As I have said, yoga is not a competition. You will have better results if you take your time.

To begin the review, let's start by just breathing. Sit up straight, but not tense, with your eyes closed, your nose in line with your navel, and your ears above your shoulders. Breathe in, pushing your stomach out, exhale, pulling your stomach in. Let everything go, breathe for a while, and be in the moment. Now let's review our postures.

Postures to Review

Perform all postures from Beginners Lesson 1 (pp. 8–12). Relax for a moment, and perform the following in the order given: 15. Toes, Flat, Chair, Tree; 16. The Cobras; 17. Infant Posture and Stretch; 29. Camel; 26. Full Rolls and Balance; 64. Sun Worship/Sun Salutation; 62. Sun Relax.

Relaxation/Meditation: Take a Break

In today's society of push, shove, rush, hurry, hustle, and run, we forget that to pause, to stop, to rest is just as important as our activity in life. We even think of "doing nothing" as a waste of time. But, in reality, we are doing something. We are revitalizing our bodies. So when you stretch out now upon your mat, forget all your worries, business, rushing about; forget the guilt you might have felt in the past at doing so. Take your time to make sure you are lying centered. There should be an even space on either side of your spine at your hips and shoulders so that energy can flow freely and help heal and strengthen that weaker side that you might subconsciously favor when you lie down.

Go ahead and take that deep, relaxing breath, that wonderful sigh of "Ahhhhh," as your body goes limp and loose, released and relaxed. Remember not to force it to do so, as that would cause more tension. The secret of success is to allow it to just happen, to trust unconditionally, as you did when you were a baby lying in your crib. No tension there, no tight muscles. You were a rag doll and you giggled! Give yourself the same pleasure now. Just by smiling to yourself, you'll feel good inside, and you will also relax your facial muscles. Remember that the jaw, in particular, is where a lot of tension is held; the other place is the forehead, around the eyes. Let's relax them now. Very slowly, close your eyes. Then open them again. Again, slowly close them, and do this just a few times, until your eyelids grow too heavy to do it again. Then you will feel even more like resting.

Now, once you are sure that your body is totally relaxed, resting comfortably, peacefully, joyfully, let's take care of the mind, which is the last thing to come to peace. It will do everything it can to distract you, disturb you, even frustrate you, if you allow it to. Just remember, if you master your breath, you master your thoughts. Master it first by becoming aware of it. Don't try to breathe forcefully, just fall into the natural rhythm of it—the rising and falling, the coming and going—yes, even the pause of it. All it is, is concentration, staying in the present moment, awake and aware, yet paused and peaceful. Content with this moment just as it is, aware of this moment, you are experiencing a part of eternity. You are alive to it, you have lived it, and you are a part of it!

There is a certain rhythm, a certain flow of this earth, and when we join it by becoming aware of it, by going with the flow, each moment becomes most refreshing. We feel a new aliveness in our body, a new calmness in our mind, a new growth of our spirit, our soul. It is an experience that can never be fully explained—only witnessed. Give yourself that gift, that precious touch of reality, of all knowing, all peace, all bliss! Join in the flow. Follow your breath as if you had just discovered it for the very first time. Marvel at how efficient it is, so obedient to your needs, being both voluntary and involuntary, depending on what we need in the moment.

Do absolutely nothing now but follow the natural rhythm of your breath, the coming and going, the in and out of it, and the peace found even in the pause of it between each breath. Doing so, you will soon sink into silence as you have never known before; a perfect stillness; a suspension of time where all "nows" are present, with nothing missing. It is contentment that cannot be found any other time or place; only in the moment where we have allowed ourselves to enter the flow, the rhythm of the earth; that is where we pause in the silence.

If our highest respect for another is that moment of silence, why do we not allow and have that same respect for ourselves? That's what saying "Yes!" to life is all about. Now, just continue to rest, following the flow of your breath. Keep it gentle, smooth, and peaceful. Stay in touch with the center of your being. It is who you really are.

When your body is all rested and renewed, eager and energized; when your mind is feeling calm and content, and your spirit has soared to new heights, rouse yourself gently by wiggling your toes, stretching your feet, and listening to the message of your muscles. Your body communicates with you when you are lying still. Stretch your fingers, twist your wrists, and enjoy the miracle of movement. Then let your arms float upward in a lazy stretch as you yawn and twist and turn, doing exactly what your body feels like doing at this moment. Enjoy!

What is our most important lesson to learn?
Love.
Who is the most important person to know?
Our inner Self.
What is the most important thing to remember?
Who and what we really are!
Shanti—Shanti—Shanti—Peace—Peace—Peace

INTERMEDIATE LEVEL LESSON 2

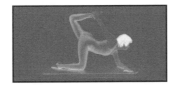

It is important to meditate with the present moment in sight. If we meditate with only the future in mind, to improve our character, to be more efficient, to guarantee some future happiness, we miss the whole point of the now.

The Experience of Meditation

Meditation is the discovery the point of light that is the now. Now is the only reality that there is. The past and future are not real. Like music or dance, meditation has no ulterior reason or purpose. Musicians play music for the experience within their playing, not to reach a certain point at the end of the scale. We dance for the movements we feel within the dance itself, not to arrive at a particular place on the floor. The same is true with meditation. Meditation cannot be forced. We relax into meditation and open ourselves into that particular state of mind. We learn to just be.

Meditation is not as much a seeking as an experiencing followed by a very quiet but assured knowing. It is seeing without sight, hearing without sound, and touching without movement. When we reach this level of consciousness, we discover our essence. When we meditate, we simply learn to open our heart. All you need to do is open your heart to truth. You're no more than a blade of grass, but you're no less than God. Someday, you'll experience this state of being, and then, you'll know a greater joy.

To sit quietly and just let it happen, to just be—that sounds pretty simple. And yet, it's one of the most difficult things to do, because of the mind. The mind keeps interrupting us with its chatter. Just observe it and go back to your breathing. Remember that when we go into meditation, we don't force it, we allow it to happen.

When you are doing your postures, remember, you are not in a competition with others. But you are in a competition between your body and your mind, and the goal is to bring them out of competition and into harmony. Perfection in postures is not a physical practice; it is a mental practice. It is the will to do, the power of concentration, the devotional attitude. Each body structure is different, so the result will be different. You are your own teacher. You determine the extent to which each posture goes. Try to be graceful, slow, rhythmic, and harmonious in your movements. Enjoy what you are doing. Be aware of each muscle as it moves; listen to each breath. Feel the sensation of circulation, of life.

Postures to Review

Close your eyes, and breathe relaxation into your body. Breathe out all the tension and tightness, all your stress and all your cares.

Always practice the postures in the order listed. Perform all postures from Beginners Lesson 1 (pp. 8–12). Then perform the following: 44. Half and Full Bow; 45. Half and Full Locust; 25. Kiss the Foot; 64. Sun Worship/Sun Salutation.

 New Postures

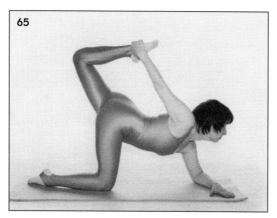

65. Raised Bow.

Kneel upright on the floor. Bend forward and put your forearms (your hands to your elbows) on the floor in front of you. Cross your left foot over your right leg behind you. Reach behind with your right hand and take hold of your left foot. Inhale and pull your left foot and leg up as high as you comfortably can toward the ceiling. Your body should be supported by your right knee and your left arm. Hold this posture for as long as it is comfortable. Exhale and lower your left leg, and return to your starting position. Repeat the posture by raising the right leg with your left hand in the same manner. This posture is a great stretch in the morning.

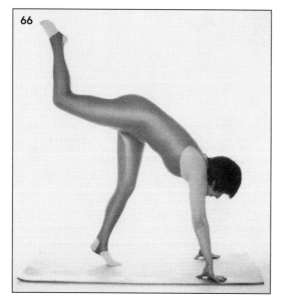

66. Forward Swing Breath (Bottoms Up).

Take a standing position and swing forward, lowering your body to the floor. Walk forward on your hands and lift one leg up behind you in the air as high as you comfortably can. Move your body up and down on your supporting foot. Don't try to use your knee to raise your body; the idea is to strengthen your feet muscles.

67. Balanced Breath.

Take a standing position with your palms together in front of your chest. Turn your palms so that they face away from each other. Inhale and push your left hand to the sky with your palm facing upward and follow it with your eyes. Push your right hand down to your side with your palm facing downward toward the earth. Push with equal strength up and down at the same time. Hold this posture for a few seconds. Exhale and bring both hands back to the center in front of your eyes. Switch hands. Your palms should rub against each other as they pass by one another. Inhale and push your right hand up to the sky, palm upward. Your left hand pushes down the earth, palm downward. Exhale and return to center. Practice this rotation three times on each side; your eyes should always follow the upward-facing hand. When the rotation is complete bring your palms to the center in front of your face and cross your hands in one direction, then the other. Let your palms separate, and lower your arms to your side. Relax. This pose brings balance to your body.

Relaxation/Meditation: Tense and Relax

Just as our body's movements are influenced by our state of mind, our state of mind is influenced by our body's movements. Our body responds to thought. If you are depressed, it might be reflected in your slouched body and your lowered head. If you become joyful, your body straightens up and you raise your head. When you are practicing your postures and you think that you have reached your limit, try telling yourself to relax. You will find that your body will respond and will take you a little bit further. Your body follows your mind's commands and believes what you tell it to believe.

Stretch out on the floor and say to yourself: "This is my time to relax. I will let go completely." Say it to yourself again and again and really mean it. With each exhalation sink further and further down into restfulness.

Although as beginners we are not yet accomplished in letting go, there are methods to help us on our path to relaxation. One of these, known as "tense and relax," allows us to become fully aware of the tension in our body, even when it may feel relaxed. In this practice, we intentionally tighten and relax each part of our body.

Close your eyes and relax your body. Begin with your feet. Inhale and tighten your toes, soles, heels, and ankles. Feel the tension in all your muscles, tendons, and ligaments. Exhale and concentrate on your feet becoming loose and limp. Feel your tension release, and experience total relaxation. Try it now. (Pause briefly.)

Try this exercise on your entire body. Always tighten on your inhalation and release with your exhalation. Practice on your feet one more time. (Pause.)

Move on to your calves—inhale and tighten; exhale and release. (Pause.)

Inhale to tighten your thighs and exhale to release. (Pause.)

Inhale and tighten your buttocks; exhale and release. (Pause.)

Inhale and tighten your lower back area. Exhale and release all your muscles. (Pause.)

Move on to your hands. Inhale and tighten; exhale and release. (Pause.)

Inhale to tighten your arms; exhale and release. (Pause.)

Inhale and tighten your neck and shoulders; exhale and release. (Pause.)

Inhale deeply and try to tighten or stiffen your entire body. On a full exhale, feel all the tightness and tension leaving every part of your body; feel it drain out and away. Picture and feel your body totally relaxed. Your body is lighter, freer, rested, content. You feel lighter, freer, alive.

Don't forget to adjust your head comfortably to the floor, with your jaws and eyes relaxed. If you are having trouble in either area, slowly open and close them a few times. Yawn, if you feel like it, and let your eyelids grow very heavy until you no longer feel like opening them.

Above all, take the time to relax your mind, your thoughts; empty out, turn off, and tune in. Your breath is there to assist you. Follow the gentle flow in and out. Let it fill and empty in one smooth movement, effortlessly and naturally.

Your exhalation takes away all tension, frustration, fright, anger, and anxiety. It leaves you feeling calm, relaxed, and revived. By following your breath, you've found your peace and pleasure, your alignment to life. You are in the moment—this moment, this now, this experience. Try to practice this relaxation exercise during the day when things begin to pile up; pause and bring yourself back to the present moment and the pleasure of your breath.

Gently stretch yourself back to this moment of awareness by stretching your toes and wiggling your feet. Stretch your legs and half-twist your upper body. Pause and give yourself a positive thought: "My body is relaxed and my mind is peaceful." Move into your full stretch and yawn. Take a smile with you.

Who says we don't get a second chance?
Each and every breath is a new birthing. Honor it!
Shanti—Shanti—Shanti—Peace—Peace—Peace

INTERMEDIATE LEVEL LESSON 3

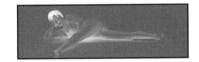

When you are having a bad day, honestly ask yourself why you are unhappy and honestly listen to your answer. No one can make you angry unless you let them—unless you forget who you really are.

Stress Relief

The next time that you are having a bad day, try one or all of the following suggestions:

• Practice your postures. A feeling of health and vitality and release will ease away your tension.

• Sit and breathe deeply. Nothing is more relaxing or more peaceful.

• Get out into nature, even if it's only sitting outside to watch the leaves blow. Listen to the crickets or take a walk. We are part of nature. Sometimes, one of our biggest mistakes is thinking that we are separated from nature. By reestablishing your connection with nature, you can also find your peace.

• Forget about yourself for a moment and do something for someone else. It's been scientifically proven that those who extend themselves to others are happier individuals and live longer.

• Make a list of positive and negative sides of the situation. Be grateful that the list of good things is generally longer than the list of bad things

• Always remind yourself who and what you are. When you are lonely, upset, unhappy, or depressed, you've forgotten who you really are. You are a whole person—precious and perfect at this moment. Stay in this moment.

Staying in this moment is what we'll be doing when we do our meditation. Some people meditate as a seeking. But really, what is there to seek that you don't already have?

Postures to Review

Breathe first and practice your postures. Let's see if you can stay in the now and realize who you are. Perform all postures from Beginners Lesson 1 (pp. 8–12). Always practice them in the order listed. Then perform the following postures: 40. Plow and Variations; 41. Pelvic Lift; 42. Three-Quarter Shoulder Stand; 64. Sun Worship/Sun Salutation.

New Postures

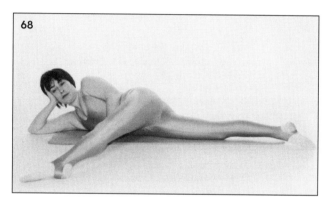

68. Side Scissors.

Lie on your right side and support your head with your right hand. Your left arm is stretched out along your body, as though you were relaxing on your side at the beach. Inhale and lift your left leg straight up. Exhale and lower your leg down in front of you and bring your left toe as close to shoulder level as you comfortably can. You can place your left arm in front of your abdomen to give you a little more balance and support. Try to keep your leg straight. Inhale and raise your left leg up Exhale and lower it down to its original position. Repeat this movement three times on your right side. Turn to lie on your left side, raise your right leg on your inhalation and lower it on your exhalation. Repeat three times on your left side.

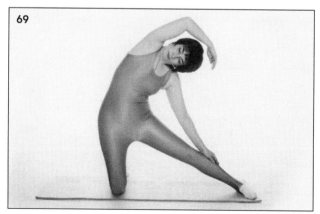

69. Gate I.

In a kneeling position, stretch your left leg out to your side, while keeping your left leg and left foot turned to the side. Your arms are by your sides. Inhale and lift your arms up parallel to the floor. Exhale and bend your body to the side over your extended left leg. Inhale and lift your body up. Exhale and lower your arms back to the sides. Return your left leg to its original kneeling position and extend your right leg. Again, inhale and lift your arms up to the sides; exhale and bend your body to the side over the extended right leg. Inhale and lift your body up; exhale and lower your arms.

70. Gate II.

In a kneeling position, extend your left leg out to the side, with your left leg and foot turned to the side. Inhale and lift your arms up. Twist at the waist and face your extended left leg. Raise the toes of your left foot straight up. Try to reach for your toe with both hands and bend your head down to your knee. Inhale and raise your body up; twist to face forward. Exhale and lower your arms. Repeat this movement for your right side.

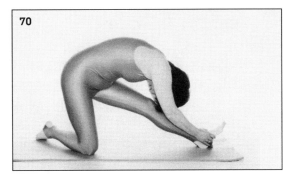

Relaxation/Meditation: The Pause of Lightness

To truly relax is to pause—to bring everything around and about us to a standstill, to a great silent pause.

Just as nature pauses in its autumn and the bird pauses on the limb, we too must pause, turn off, and tune in. It begins with a single thought: "I am going to let go!" This experience allows us to discover the essence of ourselves and realize that we are complete. It leads us further into precious peace.

Lie down in a centered position—your body comfortable on the floor. It is always important to make sure that your body is comfortable so that it does not disturb your meditation. Release and relax with your eyes closed, and rid yourself of all tightness, tension, and restrictions. The following relaxation emphasizes lightness.

Starting with your heels, imagine that you can feel the space between your heels and the floor. Try not think of either your heels or the floor; instead, feel the space between the two. (Pause.)

Feel the space between your thighs and the floor. (Pause.)

Continue your relaxed breathing and try to feel the space between the floor and the following parts of your body:

Your buttocks (Pause.)

Your back. (Pause.)

Your hands. (Pause.)

Your arms. (Pause.)

Your shoulders. (Pause.)

Your head. (Pause.)

Try to feel all these various points as one surface. Your whole body is floating on the space between, suspended, light, relaxed, and carefree. (Pause.)

With each inhalation, you feel lighter, and with each exhalation you feel more relaxed. (Pause.)

Go one step further and make the space between you and the floor grow. The wider it becomes, the lighter you will feel. This state of lightness is the pinnacle of freedom. Each time that you inhale, feel your body become lighter, as though you were floating or drifting up, slowly into space. Be relaxed and know that you are safe and free. Keep following your inhalation, let it lift and guide you. Let go and enjoy. (Pause.)

Lightness is your true essence. Heaviness—feeling weighted down—are attributes of the ego. When you release your ego, your lightness returns. Absorb this feeling of lightness.

In order to come back down, concentrate on your exhalation instead of your inhalation. Every time that you exhale, let your body slowly and gently drift toward the floor again, like a leaf riding the gentle breeze. You drift downward. Take your time and enjoy your feeling of lightness and freedom. (Pause.)

With one final deep exhalation, you are back on the floor. You are home again, safe, secure, and serene. Smile to yourself as you go into your first lazy stretch. Lightness always brings laughter, just as laughter makes us feel light. Say to yourself: "My body is relaxed and my mind is peaceful." Enjoy a full stretch, a twist or a turn, and a yawn. Life is a celebration.

Each day you should find something to be thankful for and to celebrate
even if it is only a shared laugh, a full stomach, or a beautiful sunrise.
Shanti—Shanti—Shanti—Peace—Peace—Peace

INTERMEDIATE LEVEL LESSON 4

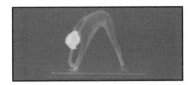

The Samyukiagama Sutra says that there are four kinds of horses: expert horses, good horses, poor horses, and bad horses. The best horse will run slow and fast, right and left, at the driver's will before it sees the shadow of the whip. A good horse will run as well as the best just before the whip reaches its skin. A poor horse will run when it feels the pain of the whip on its body. A bad horse will run after the pain penetrates in the marrow of its bones. How does this story relate to meditation? We all want to be the best horse, or at least a good one.

The Value of Meditation

The purpose of practicing meditation isn't to make you into a champion. When you practice correctly, it does not matter if you are the best or the worst. At times, our most difficult experiences can become our most valuable. Even if you feel that you are not good at meditation, you still benefit from your practice. Yoga tells us that there is no such thing as failure. The perception that we have "failed" is a step forward because we don't make the same mistake again. Instead of feeling dejected, like a down-and-out failure, we thank the situation for pointing the way for us. Meditation is an ongoing experience and process that is unique for each one of us. We all travel at different speeds and reach our destination in different ways. However, we all share the same basic principles.

Meditation should occur naturally, as naturally as drinking water when you're thirsty or taking a nap when you're sleepy. Simply sit and try to experience the nothingness of it—just being—feeling empty, but complete.

Throughout your day, try to move freely—hold and move your body more naturally. Learn to be more circular in your movements, not stiff. You'll feel lighter, freer, healthier; your circulation will improve and you'll be a happier person. Remember how you were carefree as a child? Where did you lose it? Go back to your naturalness. Now, when we get into our postures, remember that same naturalness, that same free-flowing movement. Don't force it. Learn to relax into the posture.

Postures to Review

As you get into your postures, try to flow freely. If you strain your body, you might have to wait before you feel like practicing again. Breathe deeply and close your mind to the outside world. Come into this moment, this experiencing, this breath.

Perform all postures from Beginners Lesson 1 (pp. 8–12). Always practice the postures in the order listed. Then, practice the following postures in the order given: 34. Ceiling Walk and Cross; 35. Lying Knees to Floor; 47. Bear Walk and Lower; 64. Sun Worship/Sun Salutation.

New Postures

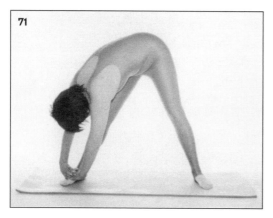

71. Standing Hip Strengthener.

Stand with your feet apart and your hands at your sides. Inhale and lift your arms out and to the sides. Turn your right foot out and turn your body in the same direction as that foot. Exhale and lower your body over your right leg. Bring your hands down on each side of your leg and try to bring your head to your knee. Keep your legs straight. Inhale and lift your body up. Turn your body and move your right foot forward. Repeat for the left side, lifting your arms, turning your left foot out and lowering your body over your left leg.

72. Toe Toucher's Squat.

Position One: Stand with your legs comfortably apart and interlace your fingers in front of your body. Inhale and push your interlaced fingers up to the sky, palms up, as high as you can.

Exhale and bend your body forward. Bring your interlaced fingers, palms to the floor, between your feet. Do not bend your legs. Inhale and raise your body up, and push your interlaced fingers up to the sky. Exhale and twist your body to the right. Bring your fingers, palms down, in front of your right toe. Keep your legs straight.

Position Two: Inhale and push straight up to the sky. Twist to the right; exhale and lower your body down. Place your interlaced fingers, palms down, in front of your right toe. Keep your legs straight. Inhale; lift your body up and push your palms to the sky. Exhale and relax your body down between your legs. Let your hands open up and rest there for a moment. Let your head relax down to get circulation to that area. When you are ready to come up, simply inhale. Exhale gently as come to a standing position.

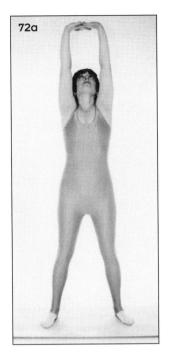

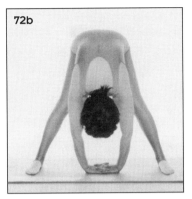

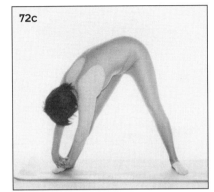

73. Jonathan Balance.

This is a nice, relaxing posture. Start in a standing position. Inhale and raise your arms out to your sides, as if you had giant wings. Exhale and bend your body forward, while lifting one leg up behind you. Support yourself. Pretend that you're a bird standing on one leg. Try to be calm and relaxed. When you are ready to come up, simply inhale and let your arms fall to your sides. Repeat this posture by raising your other leg up behind you. Pretend that you're Jonathan Livingston Seagull coming in from a nice long flight. It will calm you.

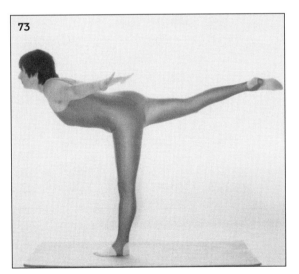

Relaxation/Meditation: Sitting Relaxation

Since you won't always be able to lie down to relax, it is good to know how you can relax in a sitting position. Begin with a few relaxing movements. Lace your fingers together and clasp them behind your neck. Push your neck and fingers against each other; hold and release your hands.

Interlace your fingers again, and press the palms of your hands against your forehead. Hold for a brief moment and release.

Interlace your fingers and place them on the back of your head; hold and release.

Raise your shoulders up and down a few times to release the tension. Inhale to breathe life into them and exhale as you release.

Reach upward with your arms and yawn. Sigh deeply as you lower your arms.

Close your eyes and make your body the following promise: "I am now going to relax. I will forget all tightness and tension—all fear, frustration, anger, and anxiety—and just be." You might want to repeat this affirmation a few times until you truly believe it.

Keep your eyes closed and picture yourself sitting in the middle of a large wheat field. The wheat rises up all about you, even above your head. It totally, but comfortably, surrounds you. (Pause.)

There is nothing but wheat for as far as you can see. A gentle breeze begins to blow across the field, and you can feel the wheat caressing you lovingly, brushing against you, back and forth, to one side and the other. You can feel the tall stems of wheat moving around you. It's a very peaceful experience. (Pause.)

Feeling more peaceful and more relaxed, you begin to let go a bit more. You begin to feel more at one with the surrounding wheat and, feeling relaxed and free, you begin to sway just a little from side to side, back and forth with the wheat. You and It, as one! Relax into the movement. (Pause.)

Put all sense of duality aside. You feel more relaxed, free and joyful. You move without thinking, unrestricted. You move naturally—spontaneous and uninhibited. Continue to follow the movement of the wheat. (Pause.)

You have released yourself to this experience. When you wish, lie back and stretch out in the soft wheat field. Let it gently cradle you and support you. Trust in the letting go. Trust enough to still feel the gentle movement of the wheat above you and the sun smile upon you. Trust to be alone, but not lonely. Feel complete, just as you are at this moment, for indeed, you are. (Pause.)

Our oneness with anything in life comes from experience. In the previous relaxation exercise, our oneness with the wheat came by experiencing what it was like to move like the wheat, to be part of it. When we learn to experience all things as they are, we understand the greater whole. Assigning names to everything around us creates distinctions and separateness. For example, try not to think of God and You— you are It. Rest there for a moment. (Pause.)

Leave your wheat field and come back to the room around you, your breath. Stretch gently, then fully. Twist, turn, and yawn. Most of all, keep thinking: "My body is relaxed and my mind is peaceful."

Smile!
The true meaning of life is never discovered,
or thoroughly understood by using words.
It is evident only in the birth of inner silence and outer awareness to experiencing.
Shanti—Shanti—Shanti—Peace—Peace—Peace

INTERMEDIATE LEVEL LESSON 5

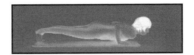

When we meditate we unite ourselves with the living stream of universal consciousness. It's as though we plug ourselves back into our original source. We gain energy from the source, and yet our ego tends to pull away from the "all-that-is" because it wants independence, and in doing so actually becomes imprisoned in its frustrated ambition. Picture yourself as a tube in an old crystal radio. If you disconnect yourself, you've cut yourself off from the rest of the radio and no longer receive any signals. In essence, by isolating yourself you lose yourself. We need both union and non-union. If the soul and the Supreme merge totally, both will disappear. If they remain separate, there is a blossoming. We must reach a balance and an understanding of both. We can't be totally independent because all things in the universe are connected. We have to honor our separateness, not worship it, while we realize that we are interdependent.

The Essence of Meditation

All things are complementary and interdependent, that is the yin and yang of life—the good and bad. Only after we sit in meditation do we realize that there is always a calmness within us. We find it in our stillness and silence. This peace allows us to discover our essence.

When we meditate, we need only three things: great faith, great doubt, and great determination. Great faith gives us the capacity to capture the inner self, our peace. We need great doubt, for we should not believe blindly. Finally, great determination helps us face obstacles and teaches us great self-discipline.

Some people sit for hours in meditation, while others sit for only ten minutes. It's not how long you meditate that matters; rather, it is the quality of your meditation that is important. Through meditation you'll discover who you are and your connection with everything around you. You'll discover the harmony of the universe. You'll learn that the unseen is more real that the seen; that the silence is more telling than the word; you'll find that the experiencing is more precious than the knowing.

Postures to Review

Close your eyes and quiet yourself. Relax and release all the stress that you've accumulated throughout the day. Let it go and come into this moment of peace and silence.

Perform all postures from Beginners Lesson 1 (pp. 8–12). Always practice the rotation in the order listed. Then perform the following postures, in the order given: 27. Sitting Leg Stretch Variations; 21. Reverse Frog; 32. Hare; 64. Sun Worship/Sun Salutation.

New Postures

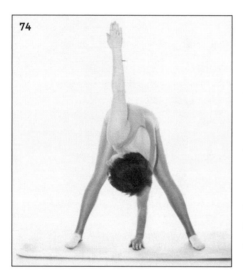

74. Centered Triangle.

Stand with your feet far apart. Inhale and lift your arms out to the sides. Exhale, as you twist your body and bend forward. Place your left hand on the floor, palm down, between and in line with both feet (do not place your hand in front of your body). As you lower your torso down, raise your right arm in the air. Both arms should be aligned and extended. Inhale and slowly raise your body back to a standing position with your arms extended out to the sides. Reverse the movement for the right side of your body. Remember not to place your hand in front of your feet and to keep your arms extended in a line. This posture gives you a good stretch. Your outstretched hands help you receive energy from both the sky and the earth.

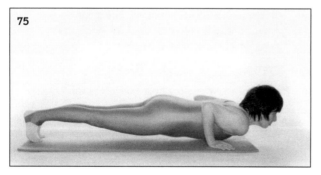

75. Four-Limbed Stick Pose.

This is a magnificent posture for developing your upper body, particularly your shoulders and wrists. However, it is a difficult pose, especially for women. Lie flat on the floor on your stomach. Bring your palms up and place them down on the floor, under your shoulders—your elbows point to the ceiling. Inhale and lift your body straight up, in a straight line, like a stick. Lift yourself only three to four inches off the floor. The palms of your hands and your toes should be the only things touching the floor. Your body should remain absolutely straight. Within a few seconds you will become extremely warm. Hold the pose for as long as you comfortably can. Exhale and lower your body back to the floor.

76. Pulsing.

This is a great relaxing posture. Stand in a balanced position with your feet below your hips. Place your palms together at chest height and interlace your fingers. Inhale and push your arms upward as high as you can, palms facing the sky. Exhale and bend your knees slightly. With a long swoosh of breath, release your arms out to the sides and down in front of your abdomen. Interlace your fingers one more time with your palms upward. Inhale and raise your palms to chin level. Exhale while you bend your knees. Turn your palms down, bend forward, and press your palms to the floor. Inhale and raise your body up—arms over your head and palms facing upward. Repeat this movement three times. As you raise your body for the third time, your arms finish outstretched in front of you

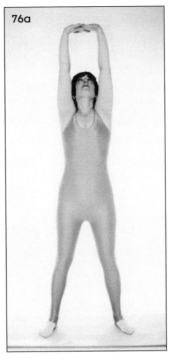

76a

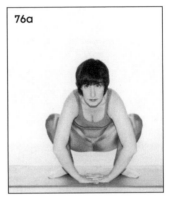

76a

at shoulder height. Exhale and release your arms to the sides at shoulder height. Lower your arms and let them cross each other over your abdomen. Finally, bring them back to your sides. Each exhalation should be a big, long swoosh of the breath.

Relaxation/Meditation: Complete Pause

As I have mentioned earlier, it's important to push and move our bodies, and to pause and become still. The following relaxation focuses on pausing to our fullest extent.

Begin by relaxing your body on the floor—centered and released. Your feet fall out gently to the sides, and your palms face upward. Your head and neck are relaxed on the floor. Your breathing is smooth and rhythmic.

For a brief moment think back to how you rushed around all day, hurrying and getting frustrated at having to wait in line at the checkout counter or in traffic. Our days and our life are often stressful, and we must learn to handle these situations. We have to learn to pause. A true pause has no time—it just is. With your eyes closed, picture a large calendar in front of you. (Pause.)

With a big pencil, cross off every date. (Pause.)

Take it one step further, and tear the calendar up and toss the pieces in the air! (Pause.)

Good! Now, picture a huge clock in front of you. Mentally remove the hands and toss them in the air. (Pause.)

Toss the clock itself. Throw it away! (Pause.)

You've just told yourself that your pause is now. You can say it to yourself, if you like: "This is my time to pause." (Pause.)

Do you feel better? You need to give yourself permission to stop and renew yourself.

As you begin to re-associate yourself with nature, pausing will seem more natural to you. Nature pauses all the time, but humans are continually lost in the whirl of the world.

Now, simply lie there in your pause.

What is a pause? It's a silence—a stillness and a quieting of physical and mental activity. It's a time without clocks and calendars, without naming and nonsense, without fears and frustrations. In pause, we are conscious of our completeness and mindful of our mastery. We are in the now! We accept it as it is. We let go and move with the flow of life. In the pause there are no thoughts, only experiencing that brings fullness and completeness. It's nonattachment that makes us part of everything around us, like a pond that reflects the moon but does not make it its own.

If this relaxation doesn't work for you the first time around, try it again. Eventually, you will just slip into it very naturally, and it will be rewarding. (Pause.)

Before you come back to the room around you, picture the biggest smiling face that you've ever seen. Look at it for a few minutes, until you begin to smile to yourself. Then, gently stretch and affirm: My body is relaxed and my mind is peaceful." Go into your full stretch and your yawn of deep energizing breath. Do whatever your body needs to do before rising.

Time is eternal and flowing. One continuous moment
extending endlessly, uninterrupted.
Shanti—Shanti—Shanti—Peace—Peace—Peace

INTERMEDIATE LEVEL LESSON 6

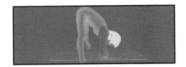

At some point in our lives, we've all been tired. It is normal to be tired occasionally, as long as it isn't an everyday occurrence. Those of us who feel tired repeatedly might think that it is our body that is tired. However, in today's society very few of us do enough real physical labor to tire our body. Therefore, it is usually not our body that is tired, but our mind.

Positive Attitude

A tired mind pays less attention to the body, which results in the mind becoming even more tired. What can we do about this? We can learn to change our attitude and realize that tiredness is usually of the mind, not the body. If you can think yourself into being tired, you can also think yourself into being energized, into being alive. If you think of yourself as tired, sad, or sick, you will be.

In order for you to lead a balanced life, you should have a positive attitude. That's what yoga is all about—balance and harmony. In our postures, we learn to both control and surrender, to reach and retreat, to expand and contract. We learn to perform these opposites in a complementary manner. Some people come to yoga as "pushers," wanting to control the progress in the movement of body; others come as "sensualists" who want to learn to surrender and relax. Each needs the other in order to become balanced. Both qualities are essential in bringing balance and harmony back into our lives.

Most importantly, you should not become mechanical when doing your postures because it will become boring and you will be cheating yourself. Try to maintain total awareness with each posture and each movement. It will keep each time new, different, even exciting. Be awake and aware! Each posture can be new and different each time because you are different and new each time. If you practice with a tired mind, with a bored attitude, then your postures will become stale and old.

You've noticed that some postures begin in a lying position, others in a sitting position, and some in a kneeling or standing position. This keeps your practice fresh and new. If you feel lazy when you first wake up and don't really want to get out of bed, start your postures in a lying position, just where you are in bed. Simply stretch your legs and your feet. Gently arch your back and wriggle your shoulders. Soon, you'll find that you are ready to get up and finish your postures. When you find yourself wide awake—ready to jump out of bed and walk over to the window—stretch your arms up in the air and start your postures in a standing position. Other mornings, you'll manage to get out of bed but want to sit right back down again. Simply sit for a moment and breathe; then, begin practicing your postures from your sitting position. The point is that your yoga practice will be as different as your moods—never exactly the same each day.

 ## Postures to Review

Starting with this week we are going to do only a few postures from Lesson 1, and add several other Beginners' postures to our routine. Close your eyes and breathe very softly and smoothly. Remove all extraneous thought. Stay in the moment and relax. Remember to always practice the postures in the order listed: 1. Dreaming Dog; 2. Lie and Stretch; 3. Leg Raise One and Two; 4. Reverse Bow I and II; 31. Lying Knee to Head; 43. Upper and Lower Rolls; 33. Forward Boat; 19. Butterfly and Advanced Butterfly; 39. Anterior Stretch; 22. Swan; 23. Floating Swan; 24. Balance on Fours; 28. Cat Variations and Stretch; 15. Toes, Flat, Chair, Tree; 18. Skeleton; 37. Airplane; 38. Standing Twist; 64. Sun Worship/Sun Salutation.

 ## New Postures

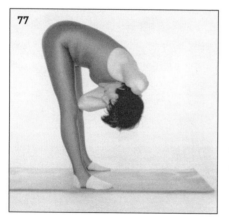

77. Standing Elbows-to-Knees Bend.

Stand with your feet comfortably apart and your arms at your sides. Inhale as you lift your arms and interlace your fingers behind your head. Exhale as you bend down and bring your left elbow to your right knee. Inhale and raise yourself into a standing position. Exhale and lower your body, bringing your right elbow to your left knee. Inhale and raise your body up. Repeat three to four times for each side—alternating sides—very slowly.

78. Standing Elbows-to-Floor.

Stand with your feet as far apart as possible, and your arms at your sides. Inhale and cross your arms in front of you while holding the insides of your elbows. Exhale as you very slowly lower your body down and place your elbows on the floor between your feet. Inhale to raise your body to a standing position. Exhale and release your arms to the sides. This posture is a really good stretch.

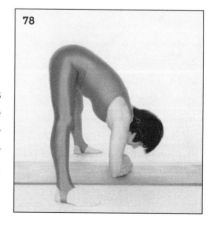

79. Standing Relaxation.

Stand with your feet directly below your hips, and close your eyes. Bring your mind to your dan tien—the area just below your navel. Relax your knees. Imagine that you are standing, floating on water. Simply experience the lightness. As you inhale, raise your shoulders and arms as though they are floating on water. Exhale and let them slowly sink down again. When your arms slowly float upward, straighten your knees. When you lower your arms and shoulders, bend your knees slightly. Allow your body to float freely for as long you wish, totally relaxed and free. When you are ready to come back, feel your feet sink through the floor and root themselves in the earth. This pose allows you to become grounded again.

Relaxation/Meditation: Springtime

This relaxation emphasizes and strengthens our connection to the natural world by reflecting on spring. Adjust yourself comfortably on the floor. Center, release, and relax every part of your being.

Through your practice of postures, you've revived your body. As you now relax, it smiles back to you in gratefulness. Breathe deeply, thoroughly, and thoughtfully, creating healing circulation throughout your being. You should feel good about yourself at this moment.

With your eyes closed, picture a very large tree in front of you. Just look at its magnificence! Look at that firm trunk, standing straight, proud, and firm. It might stand that way for hundreds of years if it is spared the rip and tear of the chain saw. The tree's longevity comes from two sources: Its deep roots reach down into the earth for nourishment, while its limbs stretch skyward to the sun's energy; by knowing the value of the pause, the tree continually renews itself.

Picture the trunk of that tree as your torso; then place your face on top of that torso. (Pause.)

Can you see yourself as that tree? In addition to seeing yourself as the tree, feel yourself as the tree. Feel the strength in your torso. (Pause.)

Feel your legs as gigantic roots—firm and pushing into the ground. Your toes are tiny roots reaching outward, spreading further and further, deeper and deeper. (Pause.)

Feel the strength of your being! Your quiet, subtle, unshakeable power. (Pause.)

Lastly, feel your arms as massive limbs reaching up and out to the sky, the sun, the wind and rain, and gather it all to your being. (Pause.)

Feel your fingertips as tiny buds vibrating with life, with the energy coming from your limbs, constantly germinating and energizing you. (Pause.)

Let your breath assist you. Every time you inhale, feel new energy enter every part of you, from the earth and the sky. Each time you exhale, feel yourself expand, pushing outward, upward, and downward. Think of this motion as your spring—your time to bloom, to flower in all your magnificence! (Pause.)

Keep inhaling energy, and keep exhaling into growth. (Pause.)

Slowly distance yourself from the vision of the tree, but do not lose the feeling. As you rest, still know the energy, the power and the peace that the tree knows and is.

Hold on to your springtime. It is not a singular moment, but every moment. Your blossoming is a continual awakening, ever present, if you open yourself to it.

As you bring yourselves back to this awakening, stretch with a new awareness and a new appreciation of your limbs and roots. Remind yourself: "My body is relaxed and my mind is peaceful." Ah, the forest arises in front of you!

Without the sun on my face, the grass beneath my feet,
the wind in my hair, the running water at my fingertips,
I feel uprooted from the source of my being.
And, indeed, I am!
Shanti—Shanti—Shanti—Peace—Peace—Peace

INTERMEDIATE LEVEL LESSON 7

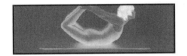

The connection and balance between body/mind is reflected on your whole person. You are as you move, sit, lie down, and stand. You are of that. For example, by putting your head down on your chest, you're expressing rejection and unhappiness. With your shoulders stooped, you might suggest that you're feeling the weight of the world.

Body Alignment

We reflect how we feel, how we think, in our movements and the positioning of our bodies. By changing your body's position, you can change your outlook on life, even by simply repositioning your head or your shoulders. When you move your shoulders back and straighten up, you feel lighter and less burdened. Your lungs will be grateful for the increase in oxygen. Standing erect is also beneficial to your mental state. If you're walking and dragging along, stop and you'll probably notice that you're out of balance. Stand up straight—shoulders back and head up. You'll notice an improvement in your walk. The position of our body affects and reflects our outlook on life.

Our body's health depends on good circulation for energy. Our spinal cord is the axis of our body and must be kept supple and straight—not stiff. The spinal column houses our bone system, our muscular system, and our nervous system. A blockage in the spinal area can cause weakness and premature deterioration of the entire body. By holding ourselves erect, energy flows freely up and down our body, and we flow more freely into life. Life is a movement that stimulates every part of our being—our muscles, our arteries, our veins. Yoga offers numerous postures that twist the spine, both sitting and standing, and keep our nervous system healthy. Our spine is like the trunk of a tree. If the tree trunk deteriorates, the limbs, our body, become useless.

Continuities

In this session, you'll begin to experience the postures. In other words, you'll begin connecting the postures together in continuities—grouped postures. Postures are grouped by lying, sitting, or standing poses. Continuities allow you to learn to flow better, not recognizing the end of one movement and the beginning of another. When you begin advanced levels of yoga, the postures simply become a continual flow—you become the posture.

In the following practice, the first set are lying postures. The second set are sitting postures, and the third set are standing postures. Keep in mind throughout your practice that there is no stopping between each posture in the continuity. You should simply flow from one posture into the next one. It's also very important that you keep the postures in the order in which they are listed in order to experience a fully balanced continuity. The number preceding the posture points to the order in which the posture should be performed. The number that follows the posture is the number assigned to the posture itself.

Reclining Continuity

1. Dreaming Dog #1
2. Lie and Stretch #2
3. Leg Raise I and II #3
4. Reverse Bow I and II #4
5. Lying Scissors #59
6. Plow and Variations #40
7. Pelvic Lift #41
8. Three-Quarter Shoulder Stand #42
9. Head to Knee and Pull #6

Seated Continuity

1. Rowing #53
2. Sitting Twist Swing #54
3. Sitting Mill #55
4. Sitting Backward Stretch #36

Standing Continuity

1. Standing Backward Stretch #50
2. Standing Waist Roll #51
3. Windmill #52
4. Skater #49
5. Sun Worship/Sun Salutation #64

New Postures

80. Grasped Fingers Behind Back.

In a standing position, inhale and bring your left arm up. Bend your elbow and bring it down behind your left shoulder. Simultaneously, bend your right elbow and bring your arm up behind your back, and try to interlock the fingers of your hands. Exhale and bend forward to create more pull. You will feel the pull along the back of your upper left arm and in your right shoulder. Stretch as far as you can without discomfort; if you can't quite grasp your fingers, bring them as close together as you can. Inhale and raise your body to an upright position, releasing your arms to your sides as you rise. Repeat for the other side of your body. Bring your right arm behind your right shoulder and your left arm behind your back. Move only as far as your body allows without discomfort.

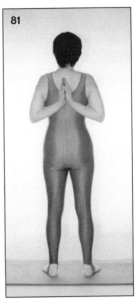
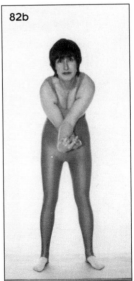

81. Temple Fingers Behind Back.

This posture is like putting your hands together in front of your chest in a prayer position except that your hands are behind your back. Inhale. Lift your arms and bring them behind your back at about waist level. Place your palms together (as in a prayer position), and gently slide them up between your shoulder blades. Exhale and lean forward for a greater pull in your upper arms and shoulders. Keep the posture and the pull within your comfort level. Inhale to raise your body. Exhale and release your arms down to your sides.

82. Crossed Arm—Front and Lower.

Stand with your feet comfortably apart. Bending your right elbow, raise your right arm and hand in front of you. Rest your left elbow in the angle of your right elbow. Bring your palms together and interlace your fingers. Keeping your elbows in place and your fingers interlaced, straighten your elbows and bring your arms down and forward, as far as you comfortably can, until your fingers automatically release. Give your arms a good shake to relax them. Repeat for your right side. This posture strengthens your wrists and arm muscles, and keeps your shoulders and wrists flexible.

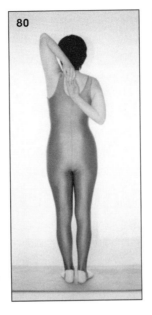
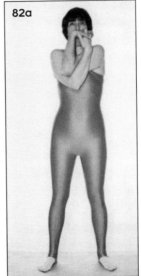

Relaxation/Meditation: The Journey Within

How much do you really know about yourself? All too often, we don't really take the time to explore who we are. If something is wrong with us, physically or mentally, we ask someone else to take care of it. Yet, those who take an active part in their own well-being are often in better health and have a better recovery rate than those who don't.

This relaxation will show you how you can better get to know and respect your own "workings."

Adjust yourself on the floor—centered, limp, and relaxed. Close your eyes and breathe effortlessly.

Every time you exhale, try to feel yourself getting smaller and smaller. This journey takes place only in your mind, and your beautiful, regular-sized body will be waiting for you when you return from your brief trip. (Pause.)

Remember to let go every time that you exhale. Keep feeling yourself getting smaller and smaller until your size is about an inch high. (Pause.)

You will travel through your bloodstream, through the wonderful arteries of your body. If you don't want to swim the entire route, simply picture yourself relaxing on a tiny surf board. Before you begin, remember that on this journey you are a curious, friendly visitor, completely in awe and interested in your body's inner workings. When you are ready, simply swallow yourself into your system. Lie back on your tiny surf board, relax, and picture yourself slowly flowing down the following the route. (Pause.)

Notice the intricate workings and the total dedication of the cells that keep you healthy—each one doing its own work—and look to really see what is happening.

Down one arm. (Pause.)

Up and down each finger. (Pause.)

Over your chest. (Pause.)

Down your other arm. (Pause.)

Up and down each finger. (Pause.)

Back up to your chest. (Pause.)

Down to your stomach area. (Pause.)

Around and around your stomach area.

Take a left turn down the length of your left leg and on the outer side of your left leg, heading for your toes. (Pause.)

Up and down each toe. (Pause.)

Once around your foot. Back up the inner side of your leg and return to your hips. (Pause.)

Down the outer side of your right leg. (Pause.)

Up and down each toe (the passageways get smaller here). (Pause.)

Circle around your right foot, then back up the inside of your right leg and back to your hips. (Pause.)

Circle around your stomach area. (Pause.)

Finish when you get back up to the heart area, where all the pumping is taking place. Have you ever seen such ingenious construction? Blood flowing in here and flowing out over there.

What magnificence! Everything knows where it is supposed to go—what it is supposed to do—and it does it! It does it automatically and lovingly. That is what you should remember. Your body cares about you, and you must learn to care about it, not only as an onlooker, as a participant. Take one last look around, and make it a look of love. (Pause.)

It's time to bring yourself back to your full size. Begin by concentrating on your inhalation. With each in breath, your tiny body, which has now left the inner you, is growing larger and larger. (Pause.)

With one last deep inhalation, you are back to your full size. Rest. (Pause.)

This trip is a realization, an experiencing of how differently we feel when we really connect with our body, when we respect and love it. Just as each breath is a new birth, each moment of attention we give our body becomes a new healing. Begin to stretch yourself back to aliveness—gently coming into awareness, Reach for your full stretch with your positive thought: "My body is relaxed and my mind is peaceful." This time add a very special thank-you to every cell in your body whose dedication to your well-being is what makes that stretch possible.

Be sure to participate in ALL the steps to the dance of life
or one day, when the dance ends, you'll realize you were only a wallflower!
Shanti—Shanti—Shanti—Peace—Peace—Peace

INTERMEDIATE LEVEL LESSON 8

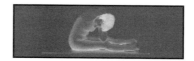

Have you been remembering to pause? Have you been telling yourself to just stop, sit, breathe deeply, and listen? Did you open yourself up to the moment? If you have, life should look a little bit different to you, a little bit more acceptable and pleasing. It's interesting, when I ask people: "What makes you happy?" I get many different answers. Did you ever stop to think about what makes you happy?

The Essence of Happiness

There are two kinds of happiness: conditional and unconditional. Conditional happiness is a limited form of happiness, dependent on things outside ourselves. Generally we depend on other people in order to be happy. As such, we are very vulnerable. We are slaves to our needs. We become full of desires, which are not always fulfilled and lead to frustration. We fear that we may lose our happiness, and become anxious trying to hold on to it. This kind of dependent happiness is very dangerous. Its loss, in extreme cases of dependence, can cause destructive depressions.

We need unconditional happiness—independent happiness without strings or attachment. Happiness is detachment. However, it does not mean that we can't enjoy attachment to someone or something. It simply means that we should keep our attachment in perspective—balanced to our being. Happiness that is outside ourselves is always incomplete—always limited. In order for happiness to be real, to be lasting, it must always come from within you. No one can touch real happiness, no one can destroy it. It is boundless, not limited.

Ask yourself what brings you happiness? Your answer will tell you whether it is lasting and permanent, and whether you are free. Unfortunately, most of us find ourselves experiencing limited happiness, rather than unlimited. So, where can we find this inner happiness? The essence of who we are is always happy. The inner being within us is always calm, in harmony, totally balanced and happy. We forget to tune and turn on to this inner being—this inner essence. We keep running around looking for happiness outside ourselves.

Continuities

Pause. Tune in. Turn on to who you really are. Begin with your breathing. With every out breath, breathe away all your fear, stress, and tightness. With every in breath think of new energy—new peacefulness—filling you. You'll be ready to do your postures. Close your eyes and breathe. In order to have fully balanced continuity sessions, remember to keep the postures in the order listed.

Reclining Continuity

1. Dreaming Dog #1
2. Lie and Stretch #2
3. Leg Raise I and II #3
4. Reverse Bow I and II #4
5. Upper and Lower Rolls #43
6. Leg Up/Sit Up #63
7. Instant Corpse #58

Seated Continuity

1. Sitting Spinal Twist #12
2. Camel #29
3. Forward Frog #20
4. Forward Swing Breath (Bottoms Up) #66
5. Hinge #60

Standing Continuity

1. Kiss the Foot #25
2. Standing Wall-Ceiling #30
3. Bear Walk and Lower #47
4. Jonathan Balance #73
5. Sun Worship/Sun Salutation #64
6. Sun Relax #62

New Postures

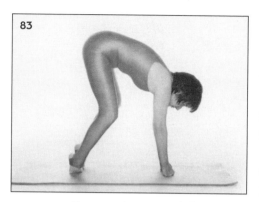

83. Raised or Leap Frog.

Take a kneeling position—buttocks on heels—and spread your knees apart. Make fists out of your hands and place them on the floor on the insides of your knees. Inhale and raise your body up as high as you can. Your weight will be on your fists and tops of your toes—do not turn your toes under. Exhale and lower your body. This posture strengthens the arch of your feet and ankles. For a greater and slightly more difficult stretch, bring your fists closer to your body, midway between your knees and your groin. Inhale and raise your body up. Exhale to lower your body down.

For a maximum stretch, bring your fists right in to your groin area, and again inhale to raise your body and exhale to lower your body.

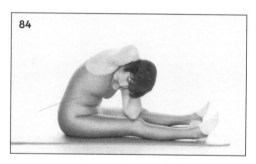

84. Sit-up Twist.

Lie flat on your back with your legs six to twelve inches apart and clasp your hands behind your head. Inhale and raise your body up to a sitting position. Exhale and lower your left elbow to your right knee. Inhale to raise your body to a sitting position, and exhale to lower yourself down to lie flat. Reverse for the other side. Inhale up to the sitting position and exhale to lower your right elbow to your left knee. Inhale to a sitting position and exhale to lie down flat. Repeat three or four times for each side.

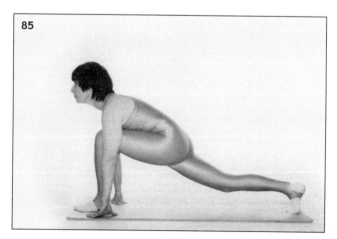

85. Wall-Ceiling Variation (Jogger).

Stand with your feet far apart. Inhale and lift your arms out to your sides. Turn your left leg and foot sideways. Exhaling, bend your left knee and place your hands on each side of your left foot. Your left knee should not extend beyond your left toe. Your right leg is extended out behind you, resting on your toes, which are turned under. Slowly and gently, from your hips, raise your body up and lower it down again—up and down. The idea is to loosen your hips and stretch the muscle at the top of your extended thigh. Repeat for the opposite side. Practice at least three or four times for each side of your body.

Relaxation/Meditation: The Forces of Past and Future

This time begin by standing. Just as you lie in a balanced position, so too, you should stand in a balanced position. Your feet will be directly below your hips—knees slightly bent or relaxed, rather than locked in place. Your back is straight but not stiff. Your lower back is gently relaxed downward. The tip of your tongue is resting lightly on the roof of your mouth, just behind your front teeth. Picture a golden string attached to the crown of your head—pulling you up toward heaven—allowing the upper part of your body to be light and relaxed. Try to stay in the now—be aware of this moment. Sometimes, no matter how hard we try to stay in the present moment, our mind keeps slipping forward to the future or backward into the past. When we miss the now, we miss life.

The following exercise is to demonstrate the power that the past and future have over you. If you learn to understand them better, you can learn to overcome them. When you are standing comfortably centered, close your eyes and begin.

Picture yourself standing in a huge magnetized tunnel. The force of this tunnel could easily overtake you if you decided to leave. In order to feel this force, surrender yourself to it. Keep your body relaxed enough so you can flow with the force. You are still standing fairly balanced and centered. In a second, there is going to be a flashing light to your left and the word PAST will light up. At that moment, you will feel a powerful force pulling you to the left. (Pause.)

To your left, the light—the past, the force—is pulling you further and further off balance. Your whole body wants to go to the left, and you give in to it. (Pause.)

You must hold your body there until the light goes off—until the urge to stay leaves you. (Pause.)

Finally, the light is off, and you can bring your body back into balance again. However, be prepared because the light on the right side is about to come on. It spells out FUTURE. This light is also a very powerful force, and it will pull you. (Pause.)

The light on the right has come on, and the force comes again, pulling you further and further to the right into the future. It's getting stronger, much stronger, and you weaken and give in to it. Your whole body leans to the right, as the force pulls you to the right. (Pause.)

And again, you must hold your body there until the light leaves, until the force that is keeping your there subsides. (Pause.)

The light has gone off, and you can be balanced—centered—again.

Pause for a moment in your centeredness—only for a moment—and enjoy it. You can understand the force of these two opposites—past and future—that pull at you all the time, one way and the other. What happens when both lights come on at the same time? Prepare yourself. Which way will you turn? The decision will be yours.

Both lights are on, and both forces are pulling at you—pulling you left and pulling you right. What are you going to do? (Pause.)

Slowly, keeping your eyes closed, lower yourself to the floor and gently adjust and center your body. Take a relaxing breath—inhale slowly and exhale deeply and fully. Let go and rest.

Think about the decision that you made in the tunnel. Did you lean to the left or to the right? If you tried to please both—tried to give into both—you probably became very frustrated and uncomfortable, maybe unsure of yourself and out of control, as you might sometimes feel in your everyday life. It is not a happy feeling. It is stressful and filled with turmoil. However, if you did not give in to either the left or the right side—the past or the future—if you remained centered in the now and unaffected by either force, then, you kept your calm, your peace. You were in control. You were the master! This is the control that you must bring to your everyday life. Try to always return to now—pause there and rest there—and live in and of it. The force—the pull—is great, but you are greater. When you realize your greatness, a greater peace will come your way and a happier you will emerge.

Now rest for a moment and digest this lesson into your subconscious mind for future use. (Pause.)

When you are ready to return to aliveness, gently stretch into your first awakening. Plant your positive thought in your mind: "My body is relaxed and my mind is peaceful." Go into your full stretch and yawn, and follow your body's needs at this moment—a twist, a turn, whatever. Then release your inner and outer smile.

What are you waiting for?
The experience of God to pass you by?
The clock ticks on. The calendar page is turning.
Grasp this now.
NOW!
Shanti—Shanti—Shanti—Peace—Peace—Peace

INTERMEDIATE LEVEL LESSON 9

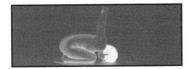

Learn to love and care for yourself. Learn to master yourself. When you practice yoga, and as you sit and do your deep breathing, you should always pay attention to the nature of your thoughts. If you think negatively, a negative reaction takes place within the body. Although you may not experience it immediately, your body will feel repeated negative thoughts, and eventually, they will take their toll.

The Breath of Positive Thinking

If you experience a disturbing mental or emotional incident, as you sit down to do your breathing, you might have lingering feelings such as hatred or bitterness. Try to get rid of them. When you exhale, say to yourself that you are exhaling this hate or bitterness—exhale it away, and let it leave your body and mind. As you inhale, replace it with love. Love will always make you feel better.

If you have had a physically exhausting day, exhale the tiredness away. Picture the tiredness leaving your body and your body relaxing—release and relax. Inhale and feel all the beautiful prana energy enter you, fill you with new aliveness. Learn to feel its rewards, and learn to feel renewed.

If you are sad, exhale it away and inhale joy. Whatever might be bothering you can always be released, if you learn to get rid of it and think positively. You can do it. You should remember that your mind tells your body how to react, and your body reacts to your thoughts. As soon as a negative thought creeps in, which is something we all experience once in a while, replace it with a positive thought. Practice this positive thinking when you're doing your postures. If you think a posture is too difficult, your body will absolutely agree with you and will be less likely to perform it. If you think positively, your body will perform positively. If you think to yourself: "Oh, I'm not going to get anything out of this. What am I doing it for?" you won't get anything out of your practice. With positive thinking, you will be rewarded over and over again. It is all up to you.

Sometimes you might find yourself hurrying through your postures. After all, who's going to know? We've all found ourselves occasionally getting lazy or bored. In doing so, we cheat ourselves. Every once in a while, when you practice your postures, picture yourself as a yoga teacher. In front of all your students, you must perform the postures as close to perfection as you can. Picture God or your loved ones watching you—picture *someone* watching. This training will enable you to get back on the right track and do the very best that you can. You'll not only feel better physically, but mentally, and you'll be proud of yourself.

Sometimes you might feel that to just sit and breathe makes you idle. Some of us were told when we were younger that idle hands get us into mischief. Idle stillness will never lead to mischief. Stillness affords us the opportunity to store energy—to find peace and reality—and to discover our true self. We must learn to sit silently and be still. Naturally, we must pause—unmoving and unthinking.

Continuities

Close your eyes. Empty your mind and experience this moment—this happening, this experiencing. Allow it to happen—don't force it. Be open to it—receptive. Breathe. Always practice the continuities in the order listed.

Reclining Continuity

1. Dreaming Dog #1
2. Lie and Stretch #2
3. Fish #5
4. Fish, Advanced Lift #56
5. Lying Knees to Floor #35
6. Ceiling Walk and Cross #34
7. Full Rolls and Balance #26

Seated/Reclining Continuity

1. Neck Roll #7
2. Shoulder Lift and Roll #8
3. Anterior Stretch #39
4. Sitting Leg Stretch #27
5. The Cobras #16
6. Infant Posture and Stretch #17
7. Half and Full Bow #44
8. Half and Full Locust #45

Standing Continuity

1. Toe Toucher's Squat #72
2. Sun Worship/Sun Salutation #64
3. Balanced Breath #67

New Postures

86. Temple I.

Stand with your palms together under your chin (prayer-style)—thumbs overlapped. Inhale and stretch your arms above your head by your ears. As you exhale through your mouth, open your arms wide to your sides and let them float down the sides. The sound of your exhalation should be a long, released "Aaaaaaah." This is a very relaxing posture.

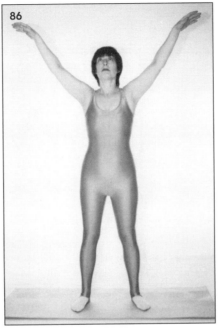

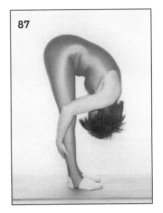

87. Temple II.

Stand with your arms at your sides. Inhale as you raise your body on your toes and raise your arms over your head. Exhale and drop down onto the flat of your feet. Bend your body forward and at the same time lower your arms and let them hang loosely. Take hold of your calf muscles and pull your body in, tightly to your legs or as closely as you comfortably can. Release your legs and inhale very, very slowly. Use your inhalation to roll your body back to a standing position. Then, take a final exhalation.

88. Upper Body Stress Release.

Take Infant pose (#17). Inhale and roll your back up until you are in a kneeling position with your arms at your sides. Exhale and arch your back forward, slowly letting your head drop back. Inhale and straighten yourself up to a kneeling position. Roll your neck three times to each side, and finish with an exhalation. Inhale and place your hands on your shoulders with your elbows forward. As you roll your shoulders, roll your arms backward and out to the sides three to four times. Finish with an exhalation, and release your hands from your shoulders. Inhale and clasp your hands behind your lower back. Exhale, bend forward, and place your head to floor. Your arms are raised up behind you. Release your arms and let them flop to the floor. Rest there for a few moments. Inhale and very slowly roll your body back up to a kneeling position.

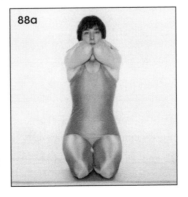

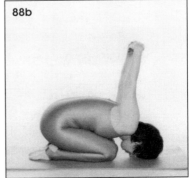

Relaxation/Meditation: Metamorphosis

This is an exercise in metamorphosis, in the sense that you will change form, much like the caterpillar changes into a beautiful butterfly as it emerges from its cocoon. Stretch out in your comfortable, centered position. Twist and wiggle to settle in. Relax your head and neck area; relax your face, and relax your eyes, as you close them and enter your inner self.

As you take this deep exhalation and let go, notice the heaviness of your body. This heaviness allows you to sink down, down, down. But you also want your mind, your soul, your spirit to rise up. Concentrating on your inhalation, take a few calming breaths to feel lighter. You are about to experience lightness. As you become one with your inhalation, feel yourself becoming lighter and lighter. (Pause.)

Only for the moment, picture yourself in a cocoon, which should be fairly easy since most of us have lived sheltered lives and limited forms of existence. It's time to change all that, to become light and fly freely like the butterfly. Some of you may say: "But I don't want to let go." Don't forget that you let go every time that you put your head to your pillow each night. Feel the same trust now, here in your cocoon.

There is a very small opening at one end of the cocoon. As you continue to become lighter through your inhalations, you will be able to pass through this opening; it's right there at the top of your head. Continue to breathe softly, and you will begin to feel light enough to float right out of the opening. Try it now. (Pause.)

If you don't succeed immediately, keep trying. You can do it by simply picturing it in your mind. (Pause.)

You're almost out, still feeling light and growing lighter, and floating free. (Pause.)

You made it! You feel boundless and limitless, as you rise up and up higher still. See yourself floating free—feel yourself floating free—and enjoy your freedom. See yourself at the ceiling of the room you are in—boundless and joyful! But why limit yourself to this room? Picture yourself above your building, drifting effortlessly among the treetops. Have you ever felt so free, so light? (Pause.)

Just as there are no limits to your dreams, there are no limits to your lightness. You can explore the Milky Way, if you wish, or go to a different planet—circle the universe. Any time you put your body aside, even momentarily, you will be free. You will know the joy and freedom of the butterfly, the bird, the drifting snowflake, the leaf that rides the wind. Look at the sky around you—reach out—and touch a star! Enjoy! (Pause.)

Fill yourself with this feeling and bring it with you as you return to the cocoon of your building and your room. Let your descent be very slow, returning slowly downwards once more with every exhalation. Relax back to the earth, to the room that surrounds you. Simply drift, drift down, until a final full exhalation says that you are home again, back from having touched the stars and having tasted freedom, lightness and joy! (Pause.)

The success of your journey—of all your journeys—depends completely on you, on saying "yes" to life, "yes" to this moment, "yes" to the experience. In our journeys, we must try to be completely aware, from silence to sound, to our inner self and outer self. We speak of silence and sound as being different things when, in fact, the original sound was silence. Silence can make the biggest sound, if we truly listen for it.

Did you say "yes" to this experiencing? The first leap into the unknown, can be scary at first. Remember that others have taken that leap before you and have flown! When you are ready, you too will spread your wings, and you will fly!

Now, in your grounded form, gently stretch into lightness and aliveness. Remind yourself: "My body is relaxed and my mind is peaceful." Then, really stretch and yawn. Put your wings away for another day and smile!

THIS moment is created just for you.
A gift to you from the supreme spirit.
Honor it with your presence by being present in it.
Now, honor the next, and the next, and the next.
THEN you will know infinity!
Shanti—Shanti—Shanti—Peace—Peace—Peace

INTERMEDIATE LEVEL LESSON 10

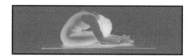

It is time for you to ask yourself the following questions: Do you feel like you have changed over the past weeks? Do you feel like you have grown? Do you have a greater awareness of your body and of your breathing? Are you satisfied with yourself? Do you feel more relaxed, calm, content, and peaceful? Do you have a better awareness of yourself and of what your happiness is? Do you understand that it's important to laugh every day and that laughter is healing?

The Five Senses

We find happiness within the discovery of our real self, and in living in a more natural state—*that* is reality. How do we accomplish this? We must first become more in tune with our five senses: let your eyes really see the blue sky; let your ears really hear the birds; let your nose really smell the fresh breeze; let your hands really touch the wonders about you; and let your mouth really taste that sweet-sour morsel of the apple. Try not to live in your past impressions, as they are of the past and, generally, they are impressions that others have passed on to you. Learn to experience your own life, your own awareness of the present moment. Awareness brings us out of our limited self and lets us truly discover this moment, this thing as it is. This reality is our true being, where we find peace and joy. When you reach this place, there will be no need for formal meditation—life will be your meditative state of being. Paradise is not a destination but an attitude toward life.

Continuities

This week you will flow through only two continuities. Remember to practice the postures in the continuities in the order listed. Flow with the movement, from one posture to the next.

Seated Continuity

1. Upper Body Stress Release #88
2. Elimination #9

3. Lion #11

4. Swan #22

5. Floating Swan #23

6. Balance on Fours #24

7. Cat Variations #28

8. Hare #32

9. Reverse Frog #21

10. Raised Bow #65

11. Gate I #69

12. Gate II #70

Standing Continuity

1. Skeleton #18

2. Standing Head to Knee #13

3. Knee to Elbow Lift #46

4. Centered Triangle #74

5. Standing Hip Strengthener #71

6. Standing Elbows-to-Floor #78

7. Sun Worship/Sun Salutation #64

8. Pulsing #76

9. Standing Relaxation #79

Relaxation/Meditation: OM I

You've already learned the value and the reward of humming. You've felt the inner vibrations throughout your body, joining the hum of the universe and feeling at one with everything around you. Remember to always keep your humming at a fairly relaxed pitch, not forceful. Let it be effortless, almost automatic. Let it be soothing and light. Remember, also, that you will experience it more fully if you keep your eyes closed. Don't worry about being "in tune." Your tune has no words and does not have to be harmonious. It is the vibration that is important.

If you wish to go one step further, try adding an "OM" sound to your humming. OM means God and is vocalized as A-U-M. The first sound, "A," is guttural and comes from the back of your throat like a long "AHHHHHHHH." The middle sound, "U," comes across your palate, through pursed lips and pronounced "OOOOOOOO." The last sound, "M," is made through your nose, with your lips closed and sounds like "MMMMMMM," as in your humming. Some people hold the first, second or third sound longer, while others hold them all equally. There is no right or wrong way. You should decide on the way that feels comfortable for you, each time you do it.

A complete sequence of A-U-M is called a "round." Your breathing in one complete round (AUM) is one single exhalation with no breaths between each sound. It is customary to start with three rounds of deep breathing, with each inhalation being deeper than the one before it. Your third inhalation should be very deep to prepare you for the long exhalation of the AUM.

When you practice this with a group of people, it is important to keep the sound, the vibration, continuous. Sit centered with your eyes closed. Begin with three deep breaths.

Practice AUM for about ten minutes.

Stay with the vibration, with the feeling of love and oneness you have created and are blessed with. Feel it with all your being. Absorb it and let it absorb you. Be not in it and of it, as, indeed, you are! Now, lie back slowly and gently, and rest right where you are.

To all of you, I say "Namaste," which means:

When you are in that place within you,
and I am in that place within me,
We are one!
Shanti—Shanti—Shanti—Peace—Peace—Peace

Advanced Level 1 Lessons

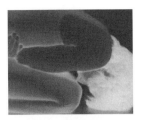

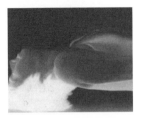

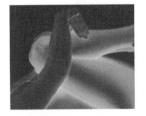

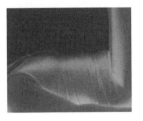

ADVANCED LEVEL 1 LESSON 1

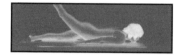

I applaud you for coming this far in your lessons! Now that you are an advanced student, there is going to be a difference in how you do your postures. Beginners just do the postures, intermediates begin to experience the postures, and advanced students become the postures, just moving naturally. Moving from an inward posture to an outward posture; folding and unfolding; contraction and expansion; all become very simple. As an advanced student, you can look forward to experiencing the postures as a meditation.

Introduction and Review

We will spend the first few weeks reviewing some of the postures we have already learned. Then, each week, we'll add new postures. We are also going to learn different kinds of breathing and how to relax more fully and advance in our meditation.

It's time to review some of the "class rules":

- Do the postures slowly

- Stretch—don't strain—your body

- Use—don't abuse—your body

- Breathe deeply, fully, and completely

- Pay attention to your body; don't wait for it to shout at you

- Wait a minimum of 3 hours after a large meal and 1 hour after a snack before your yoga session

- Wear loose clothing

Try to integrate the yoga teachings and practice into your life. It's not something you're adding to your life; it's a part of your life. You get out of your practice what you put into it.

Continuities

Perform the following continuities, flowing from one posture to the next.

Reclining Continuity

1. Dreaming Dog #1
2. Lie and Stretch #2
3. Leg Raise I and II #3
4. Reverse Bow I and II #4
5. Lying Knees to Floor #35
6. Lying Knee to Head #31
7. Head to Knee and Pull #6

Seated Continuity

1. Butterfly and Advanced #19
2. Sitting Backward Stretch #36
3. Sitting Leg Stretch #27
4. Anterior Stretch #39
5. Full Rolls and Balance #26

Standing Continuity

1. Standing Backward Stretch #50
2. Airplane #37
3. Standing Twist #38
4. Standing Elbows-to-Knees #77
5. Forward Swing Breath (Bottoms Up) #66
6. Sun Worship/Sun Salutation #64
7. Jonathan Balance #73
8. Pulsing #76
9. Sun Relax #62

Relaxation/Meditation: Breathing Concentration

Well, do you feel more relaxed, less stressed? Moving the body, quietly, gently, rhythmically, in harmony with the universe, always makes you feel better. It not only makes the body more supple, it quiets the mind. If you have listened to your body, you should feel more centered. Now, with that mental quietude, we are going to go over the basics for entering into proper relaxation and meditation.

As always, our first class of a new session is devoted to refreshing the practice. You may think it boring to have to keep hearing the same thing again and again. Please do not feel that simply because you have progressed to this level, you are so advanced that you have no need for a review of the basics. It is because you have progressed to this level that this review will benefit you. Have you ever read a story and felt that you understood what the author was trying to say? And then, did you read the same story two, or three, or even four years later and say to yourself, "Gee, I didn't see that the first time." Why do you suppose that was? Well, the second time you read the story you were a different person, with greater experience, and, probably, with greater understanding. Because of that, you saw something different than in your first reading. All of life is like that, including yoga, relaxation, and, certainly, meditation.

Relaxation or meditation can be done in any position that is comfortable for you. It may be sitting, lying down, standing, or walking; whatever is comfortable for you at any given time. Some days you may feel like lying down, other days you may feel like doing a walking meditation. It will vary—just as you are different each day—so will your practice. However, for the purposes of this lesson, we will lie down for our relaxation or meditation.

How do we lie down? Do we just sort of collapse onto the mat? No. We need to align the body. Let's start now. Gently lower yourself into a lying position, and close your eyes. Be sure your neck is comfortable, with the back of your head resting on the floor. Your arms are at your sides, shoulders are relaxed, not hunched up toward your ears. Your lower back is relaxed. Inhale and then exhale. Relax your back even more on the exhalation. Wiggle your hips, your knees, your ankles, and your feet. Do you feel that your body is aligned from top to toe? If not make any adjustments you feel you need to get this alignment. (Pause here.)

There, are you settled in? We talked earlier about proper breathing and how it can relax you. We also talked about concentration. Now, it's time to practice these two; first, your breathing. Take a slow, deep inhalation. Feel your stomach pushing up and out as your lungs fill with all that wonderful prana energy. Hold this for a few seconds and then slowly let a full exhalation out through your nose. As you do this, your stomach will return to its normal position. Now, take your next slow, deep inhalation and feel your stomach automatically rise up and out, deeper, fuller than your first breath. Again, hold for a few seconds, and slowly exhale through your nose. With each inhalation feel your body getting lighter and lighter. With each exhalation feel all the stress, all the tension flow out as you breathe away all the cares of the day, feeling more and more free. Practice this for a few more breaths and then gradually let your breathing return to normal, yet slow and gentle. (Pause here.)

Feel as light as the clouds floating along on the summer breeze. Feel free. Let go of all those things that seemed so important before you started this lesson.

Now, we will practice the concentration part. On your next slow inhalation, just pay attention to your breath. Feel it entering your nostrils, watch it as it flows down and into your lungs. Feel yourself float for that split second before your inhalation becomes an exhalation. Pay attention as the exhalation takes over and the breath moves up through your nose. Feel it flow out of your body, into the universe. Again, concentrate on the breath as you inhale slowly. Follow it, watch it flow down and into your lungs, all of you very relaxed, very calm, very peaceful. Now, be aware of the change from inhalation to exhalation.

Follow your breath up, up, and out. Feel it flowing through your nose, out, out, released, and free. You do this all very slowly, very gently, very naturally. Concentrating on breath, you become one with breath, there is no separation. There is no ending of the inhalation, no starting of the exhalation. It is all one smooth, flowing process with no beginning and no end. Concentrate on it, follow it, watch it, be it!

Whenever you are ready, gently and softly move your attention to your inhalation. Let each inhalation become deeper and deeper. Feel your body filling with energy, becoming alive. You are here now, in this room, in this moment. Gently start to move your body. Do you need to stretch, to yawn? Listen to your body. What is it asking of you? Listen and it will tell you. Now, as you come back to awareness, give yourself that one final reminder, "My body is relaxed, my mind is peaceful." Say it again, and, mean it, feel it, realize it. And smile. The universe will return your smile ten-thousand-fold.

A dance has many steps, with many twists and turns.
Life does, too.
Treat life as just another dance.
Step lightly. Flow freely. Enjoy.
Good. Take a bow!
Shanti—Shanti—Shanti—Peace—Peace—Peace

ADVANCED LEVEL 1 LESSON 2

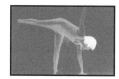

In the beginning of the lesson, you learn about practices that are advantageous to your health. Before you do your postures, before you relax. This makes you a whole person. It would be a lot easier if I just taught you a few postures, and then said, "Good luck." But then, I wouldn't be a very good teacher for you. I hope that you will learn to master yourself, to become a more complete person who does not have to be dependent on others. You can take your own well-being in your own hands and be at peace with yourself. If that sounds good to you, then that's what we are going to do right now.

You may have noticed that when you first started to do postures you would do one posture and then stop, and then you would do another one and stop, and so forth. Then I began to give you a series of postures, putting three, four, and then five together, and so on. One began to flow into the other, like a smooth, flowing river, moving in and out, up and down, around—very effortlessly, very rhythmically. Yoga helps us to break through not only our physical limitations but to break through our psychological blocks, as well. Of course, in reality, in truth, it's not yoga that does this, it is we, ourselves, applying that yoga. Yoga can only point the way, that's also all that a teacher really does—point out, suggest, encourage. But the doing is yours. You do it for yourself. So, when you "make it," be sure to applaud yourself.

The Power of Controlled Breathing

When doing your breathing, utilize the oxygen properties that you take in. Let your breath enter your nose, fill your larynx (your windpipe); let it subdivide into the bronchial tubes, subdivide again into the air sacs, energizing the entire lung and taking up your whole lung capacity. This contributes to your physical well-being as well as your mental well-being. Think about this: one minute of anger has a very destructive effect on the body. In anger, bile is secreted into your bloodstream, and your face becomes red. This redness comes from lots of energy being burned during a period of uncontrolled emotion. This tremendous surge of uncontrolled, burning energy can cause fatigue, and many occurrences of it can cause fatal diseases. While you are in such a state your breathing is out of control. Proper breathing allows pure prana energy to calm and heal you.

We have amazing inner healing powers that we take for granted far too often. Have you ever tripped and fallen on your knee? What was the first thing you did? You probably put both hands down and held the knee, and it felt a little better, didn't it? That's the healing power within you. Taking in prana energy consciously, through proper breathing, helps keep our healing power strong.

Control your breath and you control thought; control thought and you control ego; controlling ego is mastering the self. Mastering the self is to know peace.

Take a nice deep, deep inhalation. As you inhale, push your stomach out, and when you exhale let your stomach come in. Remember that when you inhale, you shouldn't pull your shoulders up and your stomach in. Yoga is learning to breathe naturally. Your stomach will automatically push out on your second inhalation, even if you had difficulty pushing your stomach out on the first inhalation. Always try to exhale twice as much, or twice as long, as you inhale. Don't turn purple trying, simply practice to your comfort level. Inhale through your nostrils and exhale through your nostrils. Close your eyes and breathe. Closing your eyes will make you more comfortable and relaxed, and allow you to go inward more easily. Put aside all thoughts and burdens that you've been carrying all day and simply sit and breathe for a moment, then begin your postures.

Continuities

Release all stress by breathing it out of your body. Remove all thoughts, enter into peacefulness. Close your eyes and breathe. When you're ready, practice the postures in the following continuities in the order listed.

Reclining Continuity

1. Dreaming Dog #10
2. Lie and Stretch #2
3. Lying Scissors #59
4. Ceiling Walk and Cross #34
5. Upper and Lower Rolls #43
6. Plow and Variations #4
7. Pelvic Lift #41
8. Three-Quarter Shoulder Stand #42
9. Forward Boat #33

Seated Continuity

1. Neck Roll #7
2. Shoulder Lift and Roll #8
3. Lotus Relaxed Posture #57
4. Rowing #53
5. Sitting Twist Swing #54
6. Sitting Mill #55

Standing Continuity

1. Kiss the Foot #25
2. Toe Toucher's Squat #72
3. Sun Worship/Sun Salutation #64

 New Postures

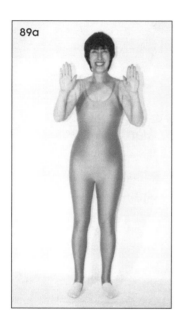

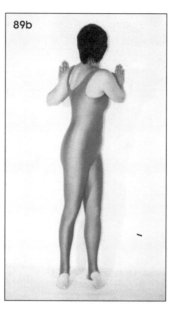

89. Wall Twist.

Stand about one foot away from a wall. Turn so that your back is to it. Inhale and raise your arms up in front of you to shoulder height, and rotate them so that your palms are facing to the left. Keeping your toes facing forward, twist to your left and place the palms of both hands on the wall. Twist from the waist—do not twist your knees. Hold the posture for as long as you are comfortable. Exhale and return to face forward. Rotate your palms to face the right and repeat for the right side. This is excellent for the spine.

90. Side Wall Twist.

Stand with your left side one foot away from a wall. Place your left hand on the wall about waist high—fingers pointing backward. Your left hand is your support. Lift your right arm over your head and place it on the wall. Your palm should face up or back, whichever is easiest for you. Keeping your legs straight and feet flat on the floor walk away from the wall. Feel the stretch in your right side. Breathe deeply and hold it for as long as it is comfortable. Exhale to release your body back to an upright position. Repeat for the right side of your body.

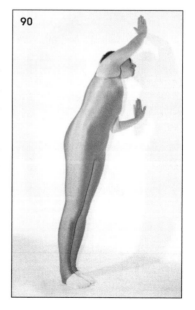

91. Half Moon.

With your back to a wall and your feet in a comfortable position, rest your buttocks against the wall for support. Inhale and raise your arms to your sides to shoulder height. Exhale and lower your body to the left to touch the floor with your left hand. As you lower your body, your right arm automatically rises into the air, and your right leg rises upward. Inhale to raise your body to a standing position. Repeat for the opposite side. After you've had enough practice with this posture, you'll want to perform it without resting your buttocks against the wall. This position is for balance and for calming.

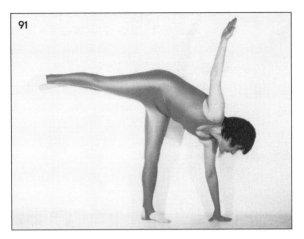

Relaxation/Meditation: The Power of the Mind

This exercise combines visualization, concentration, and physical experience, in order to show you how the mind works and how you can control it.

Lie down and, as you relax down, align your body comfortably and close your eyes. Take a nice deep inhalation to allow your body to relax more fully. Follow your exhalation and sink down, further and further, until you are completely relaxed.

Begin the following visualization. Keeping motion in mind, slowly move from one step to the next. (Pause.)

Visualize a total void. (Pause.)

Visualize a total void, then fill it with yourself. (Pause.)

Picture the color red. (Pause.)

Take the red away. What is left? (Pause.)

Your mind created color and dispersed color. Is color only in the mind? What is real and what is unreal? (Pause.)

Think of the sound of two stones struck together. (Pause.)

What is the sound of only one stone? (Pause.)

Think of the sound of a door as it closes. (Pause.)

Now, think of the sound of the door being closed with no frame. (Pause.)

Your mind has created sound and dispersed sound. What is real and what is unreal? (Pause.)

The answer will show you the power of your mind.

The following visualization is meant to help you experience the power of physical sensation.

Concentrate on your feet. Each time that you exhale, send your energy to your feet—feel it travel and enter your feet. Keep exhaling and filling your feet with this energy. (Pause.)

Now, simply experience your feet—a tingling sensation, particularly in the big toes. Feel the increased tingle spreading throughout your feet. Concentrate on this tingling—really feel it! (Pause.)

On your next exhalation, feel this energy leaving your feet—breath it out and away. It grows less and less obvious—weaker with each exhalation—until it's gone! Was this energy real or unreal? When you realize the answer, you will realize truth. Now, simply rest.

Your mind is forever creating or destroying your existence. Throughout time, every great figure has reminded us again and again that we are what we think. We become our thoughts and our thoughts reflect us. Thoughts are more powerful—positive or negative—than a lethal warhead. Thoughts are the dictate of everything in existence. Each and every one of us has the power of thought, if we properly learn how to direct it. There is no heaven or hell that thought has not created, no good or bad, happy or sad independent from thought. The generating force, or factor behind each direction is thought! Our breath controls our thoughts.

Are you in control, now? Where is your breath? Is it erratic? Is it relaxed, rhythmic, effortless, subtle, and refined? That's your goal; follow it and you will find the peace you seek.

Bring your body back to wakefulness and aliveness by stretching it gently, starting with your feet and legs. Stretch gently, moving your hands and arms as petals unfolding, and remind yourself: "My body is relaxed and my mind is peaceful." Then stretch fully and yawn. Smile back to now.

What does a smile say about a person?
That they are at peace with themselves and all about them.
Where does that inner peace come from?
Shhhhhhh. Listen to the silence within.
It shouts for your attention!
Shanti—Shanti—Shanti—Peace—Peace—Peace

ADVANCED LEVEL 1 LESSON 3

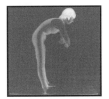

Yoga generates energy, and through your practice you can learn to store this energy. Through your breathings, as you are practicing the postures, you create energy. When you lie down in relaxation, you are learning to store this energy.

Storing Energy

Yoga helps us to break through not only our physical limitations, but our psychological blocks as well. Although yoga leads you down the right path, you are surpassing your limitations.

Remember that when you breathe, you'll want to utilize all the oxygen available to you. Let the breath enter your nose, fill your larynx and your windpipe, subdivide into your bronchial tubes and your air sacs, and energize your whole lung capacity. This will benefit both your physical and mental well-being.

Anger has a very destructive effect on our body. When we're angry and experience uncontrolled emotions, we burn energy. Consequently our bile rises and our face becomes red. This tremendous surge of uncontrolled burning energy can cause fatigue and disease, and can even kill us. While we are in such a state, our breathing is out of control. Proper breathing is pure prana energy, which calms and heals us. We have healing powers within ourselves. At times we use them unthinkingly. For example, if we trip and hurt a knee, we usually place both hands down to hold our knee, and it feels a little better. That's the healing power within us.

When we control our breath, we control our thoughts. If we control our thoughts, we control ego. Controlling the ego is mastering the self, and mastering the self is to know peace.

Continuities

Take a few moments to breathe yourself into relaxation—very slowly, deeply, and completely. Close your eyes. When you are ready, practice the continuities in the order listed.

Seated/Reclining Continuity

1. Neck Roll #7
2. Shoulder Lift and Roll #8
3. Lotus Relaxed Posture #57
4 Sitting Backward Stretch #36
5. Sitting Spinal Twist #12
6. Lion #11
7. Kneeling Reverse Arm Raise #10
8. Hinge #60
9. Raised Bow #65
10. Reverse Frog #21
11. Raised or Leap Frog #83
12. Infant Posture and Stretch #17

Standing Continuity

1. Toes, Flat, Chair, Tree #15
2. Standing Head to Knee #13
3. Centered Triangle #74
4. Standing Hip Strengthener #71
5. Sun Worship/Sun Salutation #64
6. Balanced Breath #67

 # New Postures

92. Tension Mill.

Stand straight with your feet comfortably apart and your arms at your sides. Inhale and move your arms behind you as far as you can. Exhale, bend your elbows, and raise your arms as you bring them forward to almost shoulder height with your palms facing your chest, as though you were hugging a tree. Keeping your arms parallel to the floor, inhale and push your shoulders back. Your hands will separate. At the same time push your chest forward. Try to push back far enough so that your shoulder blades are touching. Exhale to

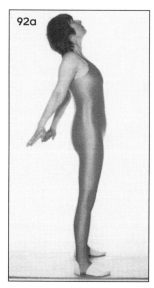

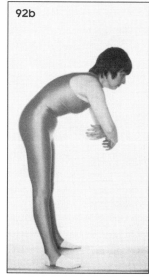

release your shoulders and bring your arms forward again. Repeat this backward and forward motion three times. The idea is to open your chest and really fill your lungs. This posture also releases any tension in your upper back.

93. Turtle.

Assume a sitting or kneeling position. Picture the way a turtle moves its head in and out of its shell. Inhale and move your head forward—chin stretching forward. On your exhalation, pull your head back. Repeat this movement several times out and in. If you have any type of neck pain, please practice this posture carefully—do not overstretch your neck.

94. Swim Down.

In a standing position with your feet comfortably below your hips, Start gently swinging your arms backward and forward, relaxing both ways. Gradually, begin to bend your body forward—still swinging your arms backward and forward. Keep swinging your arms and bending your body forward until your hands are almost touching the floor. Gradually, let your arms stop swinging. As you stop, simply hang there and relax. When you are ready, inhale and raise your body to an upright position. This posture is very refreshing and relaxing.

Relaxation/Meditation: The Inner Child

Did you ever wish upon a star? You probably did as a child. But as you got older and put aside what you considered childish ways, you probably also put aside most, if not all, the innocence and trust of your youth. This loss is one of our greatest misfortunes and saddest mistakes. In this relaxation session, you'll try recapture your childish ways to assist you in healing.

As usual, center your body comfortably on the floor—twist and wiggle—as you become increasingly relieved and relaxed, peaceful and poised. Take a deep inhalation and joyfully follow it with a full exhalation, allowing you to sink down further and further into rest. Softly close your eyes to go within.

Take a minute to reflect on what it is about yourself that troubles you the most. You might be dissatisfied with your weight or you might struggle with some character flaw. Maybe you experience persistent pain in some part of your body. Take a walk through your body and decide what it is you wish to correct or change or help. (Pause.)

Once you have chosen the problem that you want to work on, think of taking care of that problem with all the innocence, faith, and trust that you had as a child. Recapture that state of mind. When you tell children to wish upon a star, they do it without questions or doubts. They simply do it! This is your time to wish upon a star.

First, picture that star—any star. Look around at the imagined sky above you and at all those stars winking back at you. They're probably saying: "Choose me! Choose me!" (Pause.)

Once you have your star, disregard all the other stars that surround it and only be aware of the one you have chosen for your very own. Look at it lovingly and with an open mind. Once you open yourself to it, it will come closer to you and be brighter. (Pause.)

See how bright it is becoming and how much closer it is coming? (Pause.)

It is right above you. Tell it your problem. If your problem is of a physical nature, direct your star to that area of your body. (Pause.)

Once you have done this, stay with your star and concentrate on that part of your body. Let the glow of the star become brighter and brighter and let it blanket you, like the sun blankets you on a summer day. Feel it penetrate you with its warm, healing glow—drawing up any physical or mental discomfort. Simply picture your troubles flow upward on that stream of light—drawn from your body—drifting slowly and leaving you. (Pause.)

Keep visualizing the pain, the mental problem, the flaw that you wish to be relieved from flowing upward, being drawn up in the loving, caring flow of light that blankets you at this moment. (Pause.)

As those problems leave you, feel yourself growing lighter, as if a great weight has been lifted. You are feeling better about your problem. It is not a burden now. You feel relieved, lighter, more rested, more content, more at peace. Lie there a little longer and enjoy the blanket of light. (Pause.)

Now that you feel better, watch the light begin to rise up and away from you. It ascends slowly back to its skyward perch—its home amid the heavens. Follow the light with your eyes to the place where you first saw it, dimming but still visible. It you look closely enough it will wink at you one last time. (Pause.)

Remember that life is not just wishing on a star, but also experiencing it and everything! Life is being open, allowing, trusting, and believing!

Experience yourself back to the room around you. Stretch your body into wakefulness and aliveness with a gentle stretch, as you affirm to yourself: "My body is relaxed and my mind is peaceful." Follow with a full stretch, a yawn, and a contended smile to being.

Maybe we lost our close connection with nature
when we stopped eating the mud-pies we made as children,
playing in the dirt, rubbing buttercups on the end of our noses, rolling in the grass,
sliding down hay stacks, and jumping in puddles.
Growing up is not necessarily growing smarter.
Take the time to be that child again!
Shanti—Shanti—Shanti—Peace—Peace—Peace

ADVANCED LEVEL 1 LESSON 4

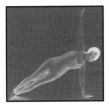

The aging that eventually, and inevitably, comes to us all can be postponed, and we can remain healthy for a longer period of time with proper movement, proper breathing, and a positive state of mind. You must learn to pay attention to yourself, to how your body feels and moves. The quality of your attention is linked to the benefit you will get out of yoga. Sometimes, we don't always pay full attention to our postures. However, by not paying attention, we cheat ourselves out of the goodness and benefits of our postures.

Feedback Sensitivity

Feedback sensitivity is the capacity to listen and understand the messages that different parts of the body send us. Did you ever notice that if you try to force your opinion on someone during an argument, you only meet with more resistance? The body works in a similar way. Forcefully trying to push your body beyond its limits actually creates more resistance and more tension. Surrendering to the posture allows for greater attainment. Our brain is a paradox that both teaches and limits us. For example, if we strain ourselves in a particular posture our brain will remind us of that pain and we'll unconsciously begin to avoid that posture, which might render us narrow and confined. Our warning system becomes our resistance. Once we force our body or hurt ourselves while practicing a posture, repeating the same posture will cause tension. Tension is the enemy of movement. Babies' bodies are so supple and flexible because they have not yet learned tension. Most yoga postures are named after animals because animals have no tension—they are fully alert to the now. For example, you'll never see two birds fly into each other because they are in the now. We may not fly, but we should certainly have attention and awareness to the now. While our memory reminds us of the past hurting, our survival system adds permanence to it. Our survival system transforms a simple "be careful" to a "don't." However, we can change this pattern by learning to pay attention to our feedback sensitivity system. This system tells us when to move more deeply into the posture or when to back off from it. It teaches us to be aware of the now—this moment and this movement.

Continuities

Breathe away your tension and all outside thoughts. Come into the moment—into this experiencing, this breath, this beautiful inhalation, this relaxing exhalation. Close your eyes and try it. When you are ready, practice the postures in the continuities in the order listed.

Reclining/Seated Continuity

1. Dreaming Dog #1
2. Lie and Stretch #2
3. Reverse Bow I and II #4
4. Fish #5
5. Lying Knee to Head #31
6. Sit-up Twist #84
7. Head to Knee and Pull #6

Reclining Continuity

1. The Cobras #16
2. Infant Posture and Stretch #17
3. Camel #29
4. Forward Frog #20
5. Half and Full Bow #44
6. Half and Full Locust #45

Standing Continuity

1. Grasped Finger Behind Back #80
2. Temple Finger Behind Back #81
3. Crossed Arm—Front and Lower #82
4. Wall-Ceiling Variation #85
5. Sun Worship/Sun Salutation #64

New Postures

95. Tree Balance.

Stand comfortably. Inhale and bend your left knee up to chest height. Take hold of your left foot with both hands. Exhale and stretch your left leg and both arms forward, balancing yourself on your right leg. Hold the posture for as long as you are comfortable. Inhale and bring your leg back to your chest. Exhale and lower it to the floor. Repeat for the other side of your body.

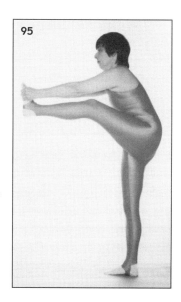

95

96. Back and Hips Rotations.

Back: Stand with your feet about six inches apart and place your hands on your lower back. Bend your knees slightly, and then rotate your knees and lower torso. Rotate first one way and then in the opposite direction. Rotate the same number of times each way.

Hips: Stand with your feet about twelve inches apart and place your hands on your hips. Bend your knees slightly, and then rotate your knees and hips. Rotate first one way and then in the opposite direction. Again, rotate the same number of times each way. This movement opens and strengthens your hip joints.

97. Plank Pose.

Lie on the floor on your back. Turn on your left side and partially raise your body, enough to position your left hand on the floor in place of your left shoulder. Your right leg is resting on your left leg. Raise your buttocks off the floor so that you are balancing yourself on your left hand and left foot.

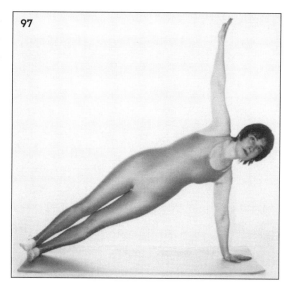

97

Relaxation/Meditation: The Flow of the Universe

One of the best reasons for associating our minds with nature in our minds is not only for the beauty it affords us, but, more importantly, for its complete lack of stress. Nowhere, absolutely nowhere in nature, will you find stress as we humans know it. Nature's laid-back attitude is fantastic! It is awake and aware to the ways of the universe and, with the exception of man-created disturbances, it follows those ways very acceptingly and calmly. Animals—fowl, fur, and feather—bask in naturalness unless threatened into changing their pace. We feel threatened and have an erratic pace much more often. We have lost the peaceful movement of life—the allowing of the flow of life. In this session, you will try to recapture the feel of this flow.

Adjust yourself comfortably on the floor—settled in and settled down, centered and aligned, released and relaxed—with your eyes softly closed. Your breathing is smooth and complete. Picture a beautiful tree—the kind of tree you would want to be if you were a tree. (Pause.)

You can see the majesty of the tree—the quiet peacefulness of it, completely free of stress. The tree is sure of itself with its roots planted firmly and stretching out in the earth—all gentle, tender roots stretching and receiving nourishment from deep, deep down within the earth. The tree's massive limbs reach outward and upward—gathering more energy—completely open and receptive.

Choose any limb, whichever one you like the best. Concentrate on this limb. Then choose a single leaf, any leaf—any shape, color or size. Let it be jagged or smooth edges, round or long, whatever suits you best. (Pause.)

Now, say to yourself: "I *am* that leaf." Think about how it feels to simply hang in the tree with nothing to do—no pressures, no wasted energy, no worries—just hang there! It's nice, isn't it? When a gentle breeze comes along, you go along with it and let it lift you. You like the way it turns you and brushes by you. You also like the gentle spring rain that flows over you. The rain is soothing as it washes over you. (Pause.)

You are a leaf—happy in your existence. You have no worries. The tree, the sun, and the rain nourish you. You are content. When the time comes to let go, you just let go. Softly and gently, you float downward on the autumn breeze. Feel it! You're flowing downward. You're riding the wind! Have you ever felt so light? Another breeze comes along and gently lifts you again. It twirls you in a circle, spiraling around and around carefree. Feel it! Feel the freedom of it! Another breeze comes and lifts you upward. You imagine that you are a bird soaring through space! "Oh," you think, "this feels so good—I'm flying!" You make another loop, another twirl, and, finally, you gently spin to the earth. You rest. (Pause.)

In your rest, you remember your brief days on the ground—the time you were blown into a small puddle and let the tiny wind-waves twirl you around. You felt so free, so refreshed, so relaxed in that movement. Can you feel it now? (Pause.)

Finally, the day came when there was no water and no wind to twirl you around. A light snow blanketed you to the earth, but you didn't really mind. You felt that you were going home again, resting. And then, once again, without any stress, you begin to grow, to blossom and to be. You allow this change and relax to the ways of the universe. Now rest! (Pause.)

As humans, we can't always go with the flow of the universe, but we can take some time each day to experience the free flow that nature teaches us. We not only can, but we must follow the ways of nature, if we wish to free ourselves of stress and guarantee our longevity. Learn from the leaf; fly rather than fail; soar rather than surrender; climb upward and claim the peace you seek.

Promise this to yourself as you gently stretch into wakefulness and aliveness, once again. As always tell yourself: "My body is relaxed and my mind is peaceful." Stretch fully, yawn, and smile into your being.

Learning true listening takes time, patience, and a desire to really hear.
When was the last time you heard a blade of grass pushing up through the earth,
a petal open, an ant sigh, a leaf fall, the passing cloud in the sky?
Shhhhhh. Quiet your thoughts and open your heart.
And listen to the music of the sunrise!
Shanti—Shanti—Shanti—Peace—Peace—Peace

ADVANCED LEVEL 1 LESSON 5

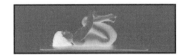

In yoga breath is often called the cornerstone of teaching—the cornerstone of technique. When you have learned to use your breath effectively and properly, you will directly increase your capacity to stretch, your strength, your endurance, and your balance. Deep inhalation allows ease in lifting the body and increased relaxation into the posture. Therefore, when doing your postures, your body will relax more easily if it is guided by your breath, instead of your mind.

Vital Breath

When your breath and your body are coordinated, your energy flow will increase; therefore, the quality of your posture will be greatly enhanced. The proper use of your breath will get you out of your mind and into your body, which creates a movement that is more graceful and much more beneficial.

Most injuries in yoga, or any exercise, generally occur because of ambition or inattention—sometimes both. *Ambition* is when we try to stretch further than someone else. *Inattention* is when we let our mind wander, which can be avoided if we keep our mind on our breath.

When you were inside your mother's womb, you didn't have to think about breath—everything was provided to you through the umbilical cord. Then you were slapped awake, and there was a spontaneous breath—a very natural breath without thought. Later you began to have impressions, sensations, responses, emotions, and your whole breathing pattern changed. It was no longer natural. It became hampered and labored by different attributes. Unless you consciously bring your breathing back to its original naturalness, each attribute will affect the quality of your breathing and, therefore, of your life. Think about the quality of your breathing when you are anger or excited: It becomes very short, very quick, very erratic. When you are depressed, your chest sinks as though withdrawing breathing. Learn to regulate your breathing, and you will regulate your life.

Breathe in harmony and live in harmony. Although you are what you eat, you breathe what you are. Take the time to breathe correctly all the time, not only while you practice your postures. Simply check yourself during the day. Go even further and take time to just sit and breathe deeply. You will become very calm and very peaceful. Everything that this world casts at you will be a lot easier to handle because you will be in control.

Control your breath; control your thoughts; control your ego. Controlling your ego is becoming master of your self, and by mastering your self you will know peace. The tempo of our respiration determines the quality and length of our lives. Yoga calls it prana energy, others call it oxygen—call it anything you wish. The fact is that with less oxygen, we are more fatigued, our mental capacity is reduced—we become very dull, and our food cannot be digested. Finally, our breath becomes shallow, and we come closer to death. Out of the approximately the 23,000 breaths you take each day, try to take most of them properly. Interestingly, most people who are tired or fatigued all the time get very little oxygen.

Taking a long walk, a bike ride, or a jog can help you become less tired and more alive by increasing your intake of oxygen. If you are outside working, walking, or jogging try to stop and hug a tree. Trees give us energy and help us get back to a naturalness. Most of all, when you hug a tree say: "Thank you for the oxygen you give me." Without trees we wouldn't have oxygen.

Continuities

Close your eyes, breathe some prana energy, and bring your mind and feelings to this moment—your experiencing to this moment. Breathe all your stress away. Breathe yourself into relaxation. When you are ready to begin, practice the postures in the continuities in the order listed.

Standing Continuity

1. Standing Backward Stretch #50
2. Tension Mill #92
3. Back and Hips Rotations #96
4 Standing Hip Strengthener #71
5. Standing Wall-Ceiling #30
6. Wood Chop #14
7. Sun Worship/Sun Salutation #64
8. Temple II #87
9. Temple I #86

Reclining/Seated Continuity

1. Upper and Lower Rolls #43
2. Lying Scissors #59
3. Leg Up/Sit Up #63
4. Neck Roll #44

Reclining Continuity

1. Swan #22
2. Floating Swan #23
3. Balance on Fours #24
4. Cat Variations #28
5. Infant Posture and Stretch #17

New Postures

98. Lateral Stretch.

Stand with your legs comfortably apart and your arms at your sides. Inhale and lift your arms out to your sides about shoulder height. Exhale and bend your body to the left side and slide your left hand down your left leg as far as you can. Keep your legs straight and do not bend forward. Inhale to raise your body up and repeat for the right side. This is similar to Airplane pose (#37), but the stretch downward should be deeper.

99. Moon Stretch.

Stand with your feet together. Inhale and raise your arms over your head with your palms together. Keep your eyes straight ahead—do not look down at the floor. Exhale, bend, and stretch to the left side. Inhale and raise your body upright. Exhale and repeat for the right side. Inhale as you raise your body up, and exhale to lower your arms to your sides again.

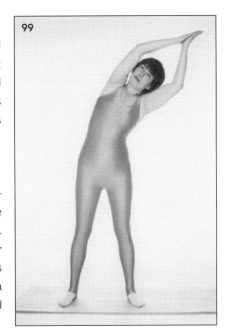

99

100. Fingers (Raindrops).

Sit cross-legged with your eyes closed. If sitting cross-legged is difficult, sit in a position that is comfortable to you. Vigorously rub the palms of your hands and your fingertips together to generate energy. Keeping your eyes closed, gently and lightly tap your fingers all over your face and down to your neck. We carry a lot of tension in our faces and this is a wonderful releaser. Pay particular attention to the area around your eyes. When you are finished, just shake your fingers and feel the tension drain away. Your face will feel relaxed. Smile!

Relaxation/Meditation: Spontaneous Peace

One of the greatest qualities we can have in life is spontaneity. Spontaneity helps bring about equanimity—calmness and composure. In other words, we are not tied and bound to a strict, unbending, unyielding rule of conduct. This isn't to say that we shouldn't hold on to our morals. I am simply referring to our movement through life. We should not always have to "do this" at "that time" in "that way." Our spontaneity should be similar to the attitude of a child—an unplanned, unstructured, and involuntary reaction to life. Think of it as dancing: We do not dance with the intent of being at a certain spot on the floor when the music ends. The dance is in the movement of the moment. That is being spontaneous. So how can this spontaneity bring about the equanimity of calmness? Movement and stillness are not opposites. When you are spontaneous to life, you are more likely to come back to your centeredness, which, in turn, facilitates calmness. Those who are not spontaneous—who are accustomed to being more formal and staid—have difficulty with the changes that are needed to become centered.

Think of a spontaneous person as a rubber band that can stretch out from its usual roundness into an elongated shape, then it can snap right back to its original roundness of shape—its centeredness. Even if a nonspontaneous person should become so daring as to stretch beyond his or her ritualized existence, he or she would have difficulty in snapping back to centeredness. Someone who is so stressed from the strictness required by living in expectation and anticipation has lost his or her elasticity. Which type of person do you think you are? Take a few minutes to think about this.

When you are ready to continue, lie down on the floor—centering yourself into a comfortable position—and take a few relaxing breaths. Follow your exhalation, and gently close your eyes. (Pause.)

Think about what you discovered about yourself. Did you feel relaxed and comfortable being spontaneous or was it difficult for you? Take a moment to reflect on how you really feel.

When we get to know ourselves better, it is easier to correct the stumbling blocks that lie on the road to the peace we seek. If you are still uneasy, not as peaceful or content as you would like to feel, imagine yourself becoming more peaceful. Remember that your mind controls your body. You can become what you believe. Try now. (Pause.)

If you still do not feel peaceful, try an affirmation. Simply repeat to yourself: "I am beginning to feel more centered." (Pause.)

Then follow this thought with: "I *am* centered." Repeat the words slowly and with attention to what they mean: "*I - am - centered.*" (Pause.)

Then repeat to yourself: "I am feeling peaceful." Say it slowly, and listen to the words. (Pause.)

Next, think to yourself: "My peace and joy is now." Feel the words. (Pause.)

Now think to yourself: "Peace is all around me, and I rest in it." (Pause.)

Say to yourself: "Blissful peace is mine." (Pause.)

Now just rest.

Just as we physically are what we eat, mentally we are what we think. Perhaps you are not realizing it at this moment, but the previous exercise had a tremendous effect on the mental part of you—your soul, your spirit. It was healing. It may have seemed like such a small thing to do, almost inconsequential. However, the smallest action can have enormous consequence. For instance, some say that the flutter of a butterfly's wing changes the currents of the earth. Likewise, your affirmations may not only have been beneficial for you, but, as with the butterfly's wings, may have changed the earth's vibrations to a higher peacefulness. If you believe that what we send out comes back to us tenfold, you should have great joy in your heart at this moment. Hold on to this joyousness as you begin to gently stretch yourself back to aliveness—yawning into this moment—to this now. Always remind yourself: "My body is relaxed and my mind is peaceful." Stretch into a twist of movement and smile yourself back to this space.

When we follow the mechanics of time, we lose our spontaneity and our freedom—
Worse—we lose our naturalness.
Plants never use clocks!
Shanti—Shanti—Shanti—Peace—Peace—Peace

ADVANCED LEVEL 1 LESSON 6

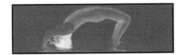

id you ever hear that joggers experience a certain "high" after a long run? Rather than being tired, they have more energy. If you haven't experienced this you probably wonder how it's possible. The answer is very simple: Oxygen is energy.

The more oxygen we get into our system, the more energy we have. This doesn't mean that you have to go running to get energy. It works just as well if you develop your lung capacity. As discussed previously, most people use only one-sixth of their lung capacity—just enough to stay alive. This is similar to running your car on one cylinder: it will run, but after a while, it will simply break down.

Why do joggers feel "high," great, or happy after a run—after getting oxygen? The answer is simple: they feel good physically, which affects them mentally. One always affects the other. When we breathe deeply, more oxygen enters our body and more carbon dioxide is expelled. We feel light and free. It is a happy feeling that we should all experience, and it's a great releaser.

Breath: The Passageway to Meditation

Deep breathing is a release in yoga also. It releases tension from the body and makes the postures easier to perform. Although deep breathing is a relaxant it does not completely relax the neuromuscular system. It allows us to remain relaxed in the midst of activity. Deep breathing also provides a splendid passageway to concentration and meditation. As discussed in earlier lessons, concentration is a progressive refining of the mind toward a focused, one-pointed awareness. We can't meditate until we learn to concentrate. Concentration is focusing your mind for 12 seconds, while meditation is 12 times 12 seconds or 2 minutes and 24 seconds of concentration. However, concentration becomes meditation when the chosen object is no longer of a physical nature, but of a spiritual nature. Concentration is a mark of genius, while meditation is a mark of saintliness. Meditation is a continual flow void of the ego. It is the merging of your higher consciousness into the universal consciousness—the fourth consciousness—God consciousness, or whatever you wish to call it.

Hatha Yoga becomes Raja Yoga when we successfully combine body control with breath control. When body control, breath control, and relaxation are combined they become *samyama*. In meditation, we do not have a thought, nor do we think per se; we are simply aware of the thought process. We just witness the mind. We look at it, we don't interrupt it. The mind gradually slows down, becomes still, calm, and peaceful. That's bliss! Let your breathing and your postures, prepare your for the meditative state of bliss that is waiting inside of you. Open yourself to it and know that it can happen. Be expectant, but not forceful. Simply be.

 # Continuities

Begin by breathing deeply—inhale deeply and follow your exhalation. Concentrate on your inhalation for energy, and relax into your exhalation. Close your eyes and breathe deeply. When you feel relaxed, practice the postures in the continuities in the order listed.

Reclining Continuity

1. Infant Posture and Stretch #17
2. Upper Body Stress Release #88
3. Lion #11
4 Gate I #69
5. Gate II #70
6. Elimination #9
7. Camel #29
8. Raised Bow #65
9. Sitting Spinal Twist #12
10. Side Scissors #68

Standing Continuity

1. Skeleton #18
2. Standing Waist Roll #51
3. Windmill #52
4. Knee to Elbow Lift #46
5. Standing Elbows-to-Floor #78
6. Sun Worship/Sun Salutation #64
7. Pulsing #76
8. Jonathan Balance #73

New Postures

101. Ceiling Walk Variation.

Lie on your back. Inhale and raise your arms and legs straight up in the air as though you are beginning Ceiling Walk and Cross (posture #34). Exhale and let your right leg stretch and fall out to your right side as far as you can, and stretch both arms to your left side. Inhale to return to your starting position. Exhale and reverse the positions. Your left leg stretches and falls to the left side and your arms stretch to the right. Inhale to return to the starting position. Exhale and let your arms and legs fall gently to the floor.

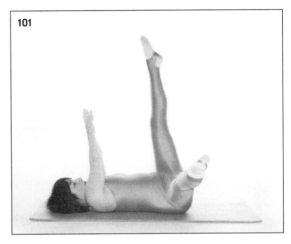

102. Side Scissors Variation.

Lie on your right side with your right elbow bent and your right hand supporting your head. Your legs are straight and your left arm is lying along your side. Inhale and lift your left arm and leg straight up. Bend your left knee and hold of it with your left hand. Exhale and bring your left knee to you nose. Inhale to raise your knee up and exhale to lower it down. Turn onto the left side of your body and repeat this movement with your right arm and leg.

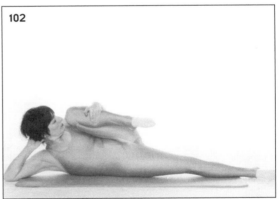

103. Half Bridge.

Lie on the floor on your back. Bend your knees and bring your heels as close to your buttocks as you can. Raise the lower part of your body as in Pelvic Lift posture (#41). Bend your elbows and place your hands, palms down, by the side of your head. Roll your body forward onto your toes to take the weight off your shoulders. Your weight is now on your hands and toes. Tip your head back and roll your body back onto the flat of your feet, and gently lower the top of your head to the floor. The weight is still distributed between your hands and shoulders. Do not put any weight on your head. You should also be very

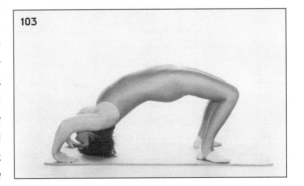

careful with this posture if you suffer from neck problems. In order to release this position, roll your body forward onto your toes and raise your head off the floor. Roll your body back onto the flat of your feet and lower your neck and shoulders. Stretch out your legs, as you return your lower body to the floor and your arms to your sides. Take a long relaxing breath.

Relaxation/Meditation: Lightness

Lightness is a great feeling! The best way to feel light physically is to empty out until your body no longer feels solid. Instead, your body should feel billowy and weightless, like a cloud. The following relaxation will help you experience this feeling.

As you lie down and take that first relaxing exhalation, notice the heaviness of your body's contact with the floor. This is how it should feel when you first let go and sink down into rest. Soon, it will feel light, and you will feel pleasantly released and relaxed. Get yourself centered and comfortable.

Let your body go loose and limp. Sigh it away if you like. A deep sigh is a good sound to the body—a welcomed sign to let go. (Pause.)

Begin by concentrating on the area of your head. Inhale and imagine you are drawing a cloud inside your head. (Pause.)

As you exhale picture the cloud floating upward, taking all the solidness with it. Feel the emptiness and the lightness. (Pause.)

Inhale and let the cloud fill your throat and neck area. Exhale, and feel that area open up to emptiness. (Pause.)

Concentrate on the area of your shoulders. Inhale and let the cloud enter that area. Exhale and experience a lightness there—the sense of relief. (Pause.)

Inhale and imagine the cloud filling your arms and hands. Exhale and feel the lightness of your arms and hands. (Pause.)

Inhale as the cloud fills your chest area. When you exhale, feel the relief of lightness in your chest. (Pause.)

As you inhale, let the cloud enter your stomach area. Exhale and feel empty. (Pause.)

Inhale and send the cloud to your hips and buttocks. Exhale and feel the lightness and emptiness in that area of your body. (Pause.)

This time, when you inhale, let the cloud fill both your legs and feet. As you exhale, they too grow light as the cloud passes out and up and away! See how good it feels to be emptied? Although you no longer have a sense of solidness, you do have a sense of presence, a sense of being whole and complete just as you are.

Take this exercise one step further. Take a leap of trust. This time when you inhale picture your body as a cloud, rising up effortlessly, and when you exhale simply think "relax." (Pause.)

Continue to inhale—feeling lighter and lighter—feeling that you are cloud. Exhale and feel more and more relaxed. (Pause.)

It feels good to be so free and weightless, drifting into a more relaxed state of being. You slowly rise above all burdens and boundaries, all rivalries and restrictions, into a state of calmness and contentedness. (Pause.)

Continue to simply be aware of your inhalation—your lightness, your freedom, and your total state of emptiness—but still feel your completeness. (Pause.)

Fill yourself with this feeling and remember it well. Hold on to it tightly, as you turn your concentration from your inhalation to your exhalation. Once again, feel that you are lowering yourself slowly, safely, and serenely to the floor. Follow your exhalation down, ever so slowly, softly, and gently. Float downward as lightly as the cloud itself, a weightless snowflake, a puff of wind. (Pause.)

You feel your body touch the floor again. Rest there a moment. (Pause.)

Do you feel anything missing at this moment? Are you whole and complete just as you are? This moment is perfect! Stay in this moment, this experiencing, this realization. This now is bliss. This precious and unique moment will never come again. Grasp after this moment totally and hold on to it, for it is your prized possession. You are touching base with who and what you really are—the essence of you. Enjoy! (Pause.)

Half stretch back to aliveness and gently remind yourself: "My body is relaxed and my mind is peaceful." Fully stretch and yawn. Smile gratefully.

If you trust closing your eyes each night as you enter Morpheus,
why do you hesitate in apprehension when you enter meditation?
Are you not in good hands in meditation, in God-conscious state?
Shanti—Shanti—Shanti—Peace—Peace—Peace

ADVANCED LEVEL 1 LESSON 7

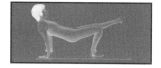

Interestingly, we often a misconceive meditation as only a time of outward silence. True meditation is silence within. Meditation does not consist of a goal; rather, it is the doing of it. It's just like music. We don't play, sing, or listen to music simply to reach the end of the score. The joy of music is in the playing, the singing, the listening, the doing. It's the same with dancing. The aim is not to arrive at a particular place on the floor. The art is in the doing. It's the same with meditation. In meditation, we discover that the point of life is found in the immediate moment. That immediate moment is reality. Meditation, while appearing to escape from reality, is really the immediate moment of reality. We should meditate as naturally as we drink water when we are thirsty or take a nap when we are sleepy.

Releasing the Ego through Meditation

If it is forced and unnatural, it is not a true practice and will probably be unsuccessful. In meditation, we sit and simply experience the nothingness of being. Nothingness is naturalness and true being. Although naturalness is an emptiness of the ego, it is also a feeling of fullness and completeness. It is an emptying out of the unnecessary clutter that binds, stifles, and prevents us from feeling free, natural, relaxed, and content. When you sit in meditation, don't sit with expectation, with a knowing. When we expect something, we want something, and this wanting comes from the ego. The real you wants for nothing. You are already complete. If you sit in knowingness and with assuredness, you will see the real you, and that is your goal. The ego is too limited and too finite to be part of meditation. Your goal is toward the infinite, the boundless, the unlimited. The ego must wait outside, outside the experience. Rest assured, it will be waiting.

You might be asking yourself: "Why should I bother meditating if I must keep coming back the ego?" Someday, sometime, these two opposites will begin to blend as one. Then, your everyday life will become peaceful and as blissful, as rewarding as your moments in this higher consciousness of meditation. The habit of anything changes us. The habit of sitting in bliss brings the tools we need for a blissful state. We cannot dwell in this blissful state without it affecting all the other parts of our life. From each cause there is an effect. Nothing goes unnoticed.

We are powerful beings when we realize our full potential and begin to have faith in ourselves. We are powerful when we begin to listen to ourselves, to explore ourselves, to care about ourselves, and love ourselves. Yoga teaches us all of these things. If we don't love ourselves, we can never really love anyone else. To love yourself means to love the essence of who you are. It does not mean to love your ego. Your essence is always pure, always precious and perfect just as it is.

Continuities

Close your eyes and breathe deeply to relax yourself. Empty the stress and thoughts of the day. Bring your mind and all your attention to this moment, to this experiencing, to this breath. When you are centered, practice the postures in the continuities in the order listed.

Reclining Continuity

1. Dreaming Dog #1
2. Lie and Stretch #2
3. Ceiling Walk and Cross #34
4 Ceiling Walk Variation #101
5. Lying Knees to Floor #35
6. Plow and Variations #40
7. Pelvic Lift #41
8. Three-Quarter Shoulder Stand #42
9. Forward Boat #33

Seated Continuity

1. Butterfly and Advanced #19
2. Sitting Backward Stretch #36
3. Sitting Leg Stretch #27
4. Anterior Stretch #39

Standing Continuity

1. Standing Head to Knee #13
2. Wall Twist #89
3. Side Wall Twist #90
4. Half Moon #91
5. Sun Worship/Sun Salutation #64

New Postures

104. Reverse Balance Leg Lift.

Sit on the floor, and bend your knees up so that your feet are flat on the floor. Lean back so that the lower parts of your arms are on the floor. Lift your body up off the floor. The weight is on your arms and feet. Inhale and straighten your left knee, then lift your left leg straight up. Exhale to lower your leg so it is out straight again, then bend your knee to return your foot to the floor. Repeat for your right leg.

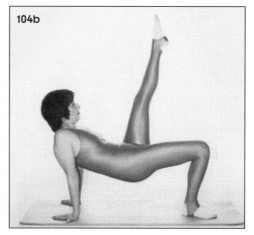

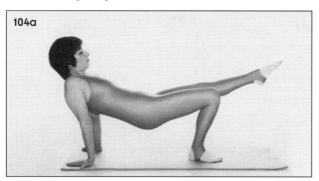

105. Lunge Stride.

Stand with your feet comfortably apart and your arms by your sides. Take a long step forward with your right leg. Bend your knee and lunge forward and down, as far as you can. Do not let your knee go forward beyond your toes. Your left leg is bent and extended behind you. As you lunge forward, swing your arms up over your head. Keep this low position and take a long lunge step forward with your left leg. Try to keep your body as low as possible. As you lunge forward with your left foot, let your arms swing down. This time your right leg is bent and extended behind you.

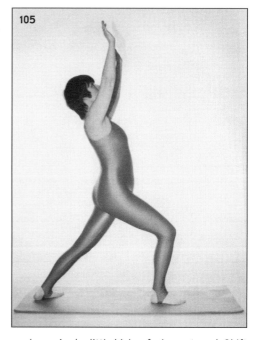

106. Pivot and Push.

Stand with your feet directly below your hips and your arms at your sides. Inhale and raise your arms in front of you. Your elbows are at waist-height and your palms raised a little higher facing outward. Shift all your weight to your left leg. Place your right heel slightly forward, and lower the rest of your foot down. Transfer most of your weight to the right leg. As you transfer your weight push your palms forward.

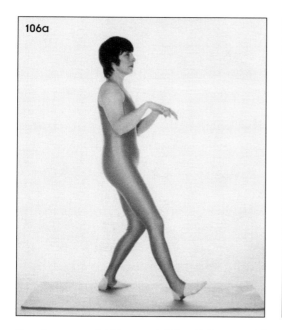
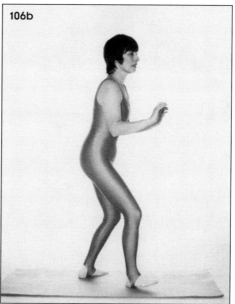

Transfer your weight to your left leg. Raise your right heel and bring your right foot parallel to your left foot. Let your palms drop slightly, and bring your elbows back to your waist. Transfer half of your weight to your right leg so that you are balanced, and lower your arms down to your sides. Repeat this movement for the other side of your body.

Relaxation/Meditation: Back-to-Back

One of the best places to meditate is outdoors, sitting with your back to a tree, tuning in and connecting with its life force. It is extremely calming and such a delightful experiencing. In this session, you will have an opportunity to experience connection in a different manner. You should practice this with a partner and sit back-to-back on the floor. Your knees may be bent if you are more comfortable that way.

Close your eyes. (Pause.)

Gently and comfortably adjust your backs to one another. (Pause.)

Take a few deep breaths and relax. (Pause.)

Think of your partner as your leaning post, as your tree! It is a very nice, loving tree with very good vibrations. Try to tune in to those vibrations now, while you picture this tree. (Pause.)

Tune in and feel the life force of the vibrations. Let this life force penetrate right through your back, your skin, your pores, to the center of your being. Be open to it. Observe, feel, and experience it. (Pause.)

Is there a calmness there? Is there a flowing and a peacefulness? Does a relaxing feeling reach out to you? Do you feel it enter and join you? (Pause.)

Is there warmth and gentleness? (Pause.)

Can you feel the tree as an extension of yourself? As you inhale, does it inhale? (Pause.)

As your breath flows from you, does it join you in letting go? (Pause.)

Do you feel—really feel—in unison, as one? (Pause.)

Are you feeling comfortable and at peace? Do you feel love? (Pause.)

Remember to experience on the inhalation, as you draw to you, and send out on the exhalation, as you release. (Pause.)

What are you receiving? (Pause.)

What are you sending? (Pause.)

Are you open to receiving? (Pause.)

Are you giving in your sending? (Pause.)

Be a vessel that opens and holds on to what it receives, but pours forth and empties out in return. (Pause.)

Now experience, simply experience, what is happening. Be free of thoughts that label you as "good" or "bad." There are no words, only gentle and quiet experiencing. (Pause.)

Remember that experiencing is the only truth there is in the knowing of life. (Pause.)

Here is your knowing. You have just experienced your other self. Now, move very slowly and gently away your tree trunk and stretch out to lie down. However, don't lose that feeling of connectedness, that oneness. Carry it with you, because it is important. (Pause.)

When I was in India I was told to hug a tree. I walked over and naturally placed my arms around it as though hugging a person. I was very quickly informed that I was doing it the wrong way. Instead, I was told to stand with my back to the tree and reach my arms backward to hug it. At first, I did not understand why. I even felt a little awkward and foolish. I feel grateful to have bowed to try this new experience. It helped change my life, and I've never forgotten that moment.

Perhaps you feel foolish sometimes in the things you are asked to do in this book. That's understandable. You are right to ask questions rather than to follow blindly. That is most wise, and you should continue to question. However, unless you try new things, even what seems strange, there is no growth. We are here to learn, to grow, to become. You must do this for yourself. No teacher, however good, can do it for you. Teachers are here to lead you. The goal should always be to become your own self-master, independent of any teacher. You should remember this lesson when others tell you that you should forever follow. Know you can do it.

Be restful, but aware. Be silent, but hear. Say nothing, yet speak. Unmoving, feel life. Unsmiling, be happy. Live in immortality—now!

It is time to wake yourself back to aliveness. Beginning with a half stretch, then fully stretch, as you affirm: "My body is relaxed and my mind is peaceful." Release a big yawn, and smile happily. Welcome home!

If you remember Who and What you are,
there is no aloneness in your life.
You are connected!
Shanti—Shanti—Shanti—Peace—Peace—Peace

ADVANCED LEVEL 1 LESSON 8

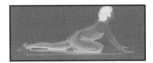

Concentration is often defined as thoughtful, while meditation is considered deep thought. These definitions, however, are rather limited. Concentration wanders, and meditation investigates. Concentration rises from intelligence, and meditation rises from reason. Concentration sheds the light of a single ray upon innumerable objects, while meditation's persevering intent is on one thing only. Concentration wanders in clear truths, and meditation seeks out what is hidden. One could say that concentration is a ray of light and meditation is a laser beam. Both help us see; but one provides more clarity. They are different entities, with different purposes. Concentration is beneficial, calming, and restful. It allows us to grow. Meditation unlocks the prison and loosens the chains of self. It restores us to our birthright, and reunites our self with the living stream of universal consciousness and creativeness. Meditation is a most concentrated thought, yet it is really not thought but a state of being. It is Self—the real Self—the inner Self.

Why Should You Meditate?

We must try to reach the highest mental and spiritual state attainable to us. We spend most of our time obtaining materialistic things, but very little time at all attaining our mental and spiritual growth. The materialistic world is fleeting, with limited pleasures and value. The spiritual realm is constant and priceless, with unlimited pleasures, unlimited peace, and unlimited presence. The material world is expensive, the place of spirit is free. You simply have to open yourself to it, as the flower opens itself trustingly, as the bird flies assuredly, as the tree bends lovingly to its true potential.

This journey means that we must draw on resources that we generally leave undeveloped. Work to be quiet. Empty your mind. Open your heart. Recognize the oneness of all. Truly desire a higher consciousness. Strive to be free of desire for reward or gain, free of preconceived ideas of reality. Learn to just be here now. Remember that meditation is the total experience of now, as is enlightenment.

Continuities

Sit with your eyes closed and begin your breathing. Adjust your body comfortably, and think about your breath—experience it deeply. As you exhale, you will relax. Let go further and further, and further. Simply relax with each exhalation. When you're ready to begin, practice the postures in the continuities in the order listed.

Standing Continuity

1. Standing Backward Stretch
2. Tension Mill #92
3. Back and Hips Rotations #96
4. Standing Hip Strengthener #71 #50
5. Wall-Ceiling Variation #85
6. Standing Wall-Ceiling #30
7. Sun Worship/Sun Salutation #64
8. Sun Relax #62

Reclining Continuity

1. Fish #5
2. Leg Raise I and II #3
3. Upper and Lower Rolls #43
4. Leg Up/Sit Up #63
5. Instant Corpse #58

Reclining/Seated Continuity

1. Reverse Balance Leg Lift #104
2. Lotus Relaxed Posture #57
3. Shoulder Lift and Roll #8
4. Neck Roll #7
5. Lion #11

New Postures

107. Infant—Palms Down Stretch.

Start in Infant pose (#17). Bring your arms in front of you with the palms of your hands on the floor. Stretch your left leg out behind you as far as you can. Inhale and push down with your palms, and raise your head and body slightly. Fully stretch your arms and your extended leg. Exhale and return your left

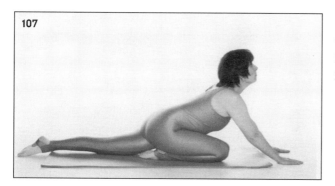

107

leg to its kneeling position. Inhale and repeat this movement, extending your right leg. Exhale and return to your starting position.

108. Infant—Arms Up Back Stretch.

Start in the Infant pose (#17). Stretch your left leg out behind you as far as you can. Inhale and raise your upper body. Stretch your arms out behind you and arch your back. Tip your head back to look at the ceiling. Exhale to lower your upper body down, and return your leg to the kneeling position. Inhale and repeat the posture for your right leg.

109. Circle Earth/Gather Clouds (relax).

Stand in a relaxed position and slowly let your upper body bend forward until your hands almost touch the floor. If you are really relaxed, your arms will feel as though they are not attached to your body, and they

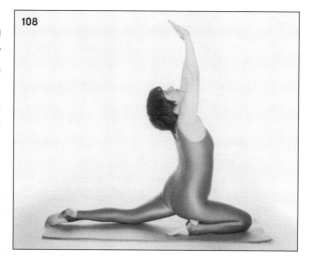

108

will begin to slowly move in circles—clockwise for your left arm and counterclockwise for your right arm. Relax your knees and begin swaying back and forth. Your arms will swing out into larger and larger circles, overlapping one another and circling the earth. Keeping your body swaying naturally, gradually rise up. Keep your arms hanging loosely and making circles. Gradually move your arms over your head, making circles as though you were gathering clouds in your arms and into your being. Then, gradually lower your body again with your arms still loosely circling. Slowly, stop swaying. Your arms will slow down to small circles. To raise your body, simply take a deep inhalation. Your arms will stop swinging, and your body will rise and be relaxed.

Relaxation/Meditation: The Four Elements

There must have been a time in your life when you gazed upon a Japanese garden and thought: "How beautiful." Japanese gardens are laid out in the same relationship as a person's body. For example, the water represents the flow of our blood, the rocks mirror our bones, the moss is our skin, and so on. The Japanese feel more connected to nature than most Westerners. We are missing out on a very valuable asset in helping us relieve our stress and in reaching the calm we need. In Japan you will see entire families spending hours sitting on the porch, gazing at beds of raked stones and islands of larger rocks. We must not fail take the time to connect with nature.

This relaxation will help you become more attuned to the nature within you. You will learn how you can associate with it more closely. You'll experience the different elements of nature as a part of you.

Place yourself in a relaxed, centered position on the floor. Breathe yourself into a relaxed state of being with a full exhalation, maybe a sigh, as you let go, or even an inner affirmation, such as: "I now open myself to this moment, this experiencing, for this is my time to just let go." Then, do it. (Pause.)

The four elements are: air, earth, fire, and water. Begin with water. It might be easier to associate with water since our body is about 75 percent water—sweat, tears, blood. We sometimes feel the pull of the moon, much like its pull on the ocean tides. Perhaps, as some believe, this is because our beginning, eons ago, was in the oceans. Water is our friend. It is second only to oxygen in energizing our body. As we relax, it supports us, whether in the tub, a pond, a river, or an ocean. Try to connect with it now. Picture yourself relaxing on any body of water you choose. Feel the buoyancy. Feel yourself floating. If you are on the ocean, feel the up and down swell as the waves gently and softly lift you. Experience it! (Pause here.)

Let us go to earth, which is the denseness of you. Feel that denseness now. Realize the significance of the way that your body feels to the floor. Think of how the earth supplies you with the foods you need and how it nourishes you. Our intake of the earth's nourishment allows our bodies to build new cells that give us a whole new body every seven years. Our excess leaves the body to return to the earth, to be reformed and returned again and again, until we too become a part of the earth. We are no longer separate, but joined as one. Picture yourself standing on the earth, pushing your toes deep into the crust of the soil, rooting yourself. Feel the rough and the smooth of it, the warmth of it, the life within it. (Pause.)

Look at air—oxygen. In yoga air is known as prana energy. Prana energy is what is sustaining you right now. Even when you pay no heed, it supports you and gives you life! Every time that you inhale your cells become awake and come to life. Every time you exhale a part of you goes out into the universe, recycling again and again. It has been said that we may well be breathing in the recycled breath of those from long ago, from Plato to Beethoven, from Peter the Great to Joan of Arc, from the jungle gorilla to the desert fox. Likewise, in time, our breath will return again and again, somewhat changed, but still a part of us. Who or what are you inhaling now? Can you really feel the energy of that breath? Experience it! (Pause.)

Come to fire. You may ask: "What does that have to do with me?" Have you never felt the warmth of the sun penetrate deep within you? Is not your inner metabolism a form of fire, heat, energy? Your breathing creates within you the fire that sustains you, just as the sun sustains plant life and warms the earth, and energizes the universe. Picture yourself lying on a warm beach. With each inhalation feel the warmth being drawn into your body, not hot but comforting and warm. When we try to understand our partnership with the world of nature around us—our precious interconnectedness—then, we begin to respect it and give it the attention it so desperately needs and deserves.

As an earth person—a universal being and a nature lover—stretch! Gently remind yourself: "My body is relaxed and my mind is peaceful." Stretch fully, yawn with comfort, and smile gratefully.

Trees offer us cool shade from the summer sun, and we repay them by cutting off their limbs.
They give us oxygen to breath, and we repay them with poisonous sprays.
It is no wonder that they stand with their limbs raised toward the heavens
as though praying for help.
Shanti—Shanti—Shanti—Peace—Peace—Peace

ADVANCED LEVEL 1 LESSON 9

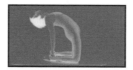

A sixth-century master said that meditation is the practice of mind control by which we stop all thinking and seek to realize truth in its essence. Realizing truth, or as I prefer to think of it, discovering truth, is one of the advantages of meditation. Most of us believe that we know what truth is, just as surely as we believe in the truth of a dream. However, when we awaken, we discover that the dream was not real. Truth is like that fleeting dream. We believe that we understand it now, in this state of mind, but we can't know truth. This state of mind is clouded and distorted by the impressions of the ego, by names, titles, and descriptions. We accept all this as "truth." But what we are really faced with is classification, not truth itself. Our classifications are clumped as: "good and bad," "beautiful and ugly," "big and small," "thin and fat," "pleasure and pain," and so on. They are all just impressions of what is, not as it is, in the same way that "looking" is not necessarily "seeing" (and usually isn't).

The Essence of Truth

When we bypass the ego and rid ourselves of its impressions and classifications, we see things in their pure and real glory, things as they are. The is-ness, the such-ness comes through untarnished, unchanged in total reality.

Another master once said that we should not seek the truth, but only cease thinking in distinctions. In other words, if we keep making distinctions, we will never find truth and, without truth, we are living a lie.

Our five senses—sight, hearing, taste, touch, and smell—know truth. We often do not open ourselves to their messages. We add to them. For example, our eyes see only color and form. On the other hand, we, the ego, put a name to it. Our ears hear only sounds and vibrations. We name these sounds.

You might ask: "Shall we go back to never naming anything?" Of course not. In our everyday society, we need names, labels, and titles. However, wouldn't you truly like to see everything as it really is? Wouldn't you like to know what "blue" is? What "sky" is? What "stones" and "stars" are? How "grass" feels without any preconception? It is like looking out of the window through a curtain, until, one day, you push the curtain aside and really see.

Once, in the early morning, I was going for a walk with my dog. It had rained the night before. We hadn't walked very far when my dog suddenly stopped to smell something. I looked down at my feet, and saw something that I had never seen before. I cannot even describe what I saw because there are no words for it. It was absolutely indescribable and magnificent. I stood in awe of this sight. It was a feeling I had never had before. My dog finished "doing his thing," and we moved on. I kept trying to review in my brain, in my mind, in my seeing, what I had just witnessed. I continued doing this for the full hour that we walked. As we headed back home, we went by the exact spot where we first stopped. I looked down again and the only thing there was a circle of small wet rocks, resembling shiny little diamonds. This time, however, my ego was looking, not seeing, and I named my impression of what was on the ground below me. Of course, it wasn't nearly as beautiful, not nearly as magnificent, only a bunch of dampened pebbles. One of the rewards of being in yoga is that this type of experience occurs every so often. When we least expect it, we really see something. It's like being born at this moment, like taking the first step into this world, and really seeing it untarnished, untainted as it is. Those brief moments are simply magnificent. They are unexpected, unplanned, and unforgettable.

Continuities

Close your eyes and breathe into relaxation. Then practice the postures in the following continuities in the order listed.

Seated Continuity

1. Fingers (Raindrops) #100
2. Neck Roll #7
3. Turtle #93
4 Shoulder Lift and Roll #8
5. Sitting Backward Stretch #36
6. Rowing #53
7. Sitting Twist Swing #54
8. Sitting Mill #55

Reclining Continuity

1. Swan #22
2. Floating Swan #23
3. Balance on Fours #24
4. Cat Variations and Stretch #28
5. Hinge #60
6. Hare #32

Standing Continuity

1. Airplane #37
2. Standing Twist #38
3. Kiss the Foot #25
4. Sun Worship/Sun Salutation #64

 New Postures

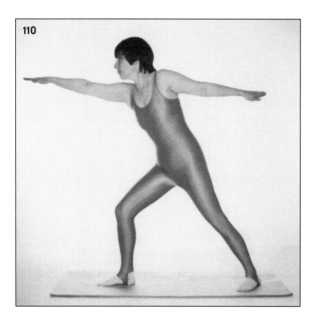

110. Warrior.

Stand with your feet about four feet apart, or as far as it is comfortable for you. Your arms are out straight to the side at shoulder height. Turn your left leg and left foot slightly inward. Turn your right leg and right foot slightly outward. Be sure to turn from your hip, not from your knee. Do not twist your knee. Your right heel should be in line with your left heel, and your body faces forward. Bend your right knee and lunge down to the right. Your knee should not extend beyond your right toes. Keep your left leg straight. Turn your head to look over your right leg. Hold this position for about six breaths, or as long as you are comfortable. Return to the starting position and repeat the posture for your left leg. This posture should be performed at least three times for each side.

111. Standing Wing.

Stand in a comfortable position with your eyes closed. Feel rooted in your feet. Feel your body light and relaxed. Your arms are free at your sides, light and flowing, like huge wings hanging down. Imagine that a slight breeze moves them back and forth, very lightly, carefree, relaxed, and peaceful. The more relaxed you are, the freer you are. The freer your arms feel, the more calm you become inside. Simply imagine that wind pulling on the huge wings that were once your arms. Relax.

112. Wheel.

This is an advanced Camel position and has two variations.

First Variation: Take the same kneeling position as Camel (#29). Sit on your knees with your feet stretched out on the floor, and place your hands on the floor behind you. Lift up your pelvic area, lean backward, and place your hands on your ankles. Inhale and lift your midsection upward and outward. Exhale and lower your body down.

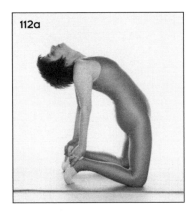
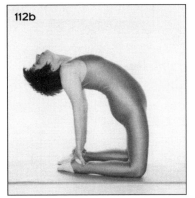
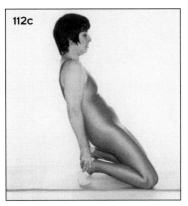

Second Variation: Take the same kneeling position as in the first variation, except that this time you'll want to keep your feet flat on the floor (see 112b). Lean back and place your hands on your ankles. Inhale to lift your midsection and exhale to lower it down.

If you'd like a more challenging posture, assume the above kneeling position, sit on your heels, and place your hands on your ankles. Inhale and lift your body up into the position and exhale to lower yourself.

Relaxation/Meditation: Connecting with the Inner Self

Our biggest enemy is usually our ego. It can possess us, control us, dominate us, rule us, captivate us, and ruin us! It is very powerful. Should we do away with it? Should we even go so far as to kill it? No. The ego is very useful for operating in our everyday world. We can learn to live with it if—and this is a very big if—we are the master of our ego and do not allow it to be the master of us. The following relaxation will help you more fully understand this concept.

Make yourself comfortable on the floor. Stretch out in your usual centered position with your body released and relaxed on the floor. Gently close your eyes and breathe smoothly and effortlessly.

With your eyes closed, picture yourself—what you think you are. Clearly picture every detail of your face. (Pause.)

It's not easy, is it? It's not clear at all. It's fuzzy and blurred. You can't really get a clear picture, can you? The more you try to see it, the more frustrated you become. It's evading you. You grow uneasy. You grow. Relax a moment, and try it again. (Pause.)

Perhaps, you see only a rough outline. When your eyes are open, you are so sure that it exists, that it is so real, but now you can't even *see* it. Maybe it's dead. Keeping your eyes closed, picture yourself dead. (Pause.)

You're frowning, again, and your breathing is becoming uneasy. You're not a bit comfortable, are you? The problem is this: the ego will never let you picture it dead. Always remember the elusiveness of this thing you cling to so tightly. Remember also how very uncomfortable you felt when you concentrated on it. There is a reason for this uneasiness. You cannot meditate on the "I," the ego, the small "self." All must wait outside when you go inside to the inner self. That inner being is waiting to greet you, simply listen to what it is saying to you. Try to feel the words as you totally open yourself, released and relaxed, to this moment, this tuning in and turning on to what it is saying to you. (Pause.)

Your inner self is telling you to come home, to come back to your source. (Pause.)

It is saying that it has waited a long time for you to reconnect. (Pause.)

It welcomes you warmly. Can you feel that warmth? It's as if someone has just covered you with a soft blanket, making you feel all cozy and calm. Feel it. (Pause.)

Isn't it good to be home again, and received so warmly? (Pause.)

Bask in that warmth, in that radiating love you feel filling you. (Pause.)

You are feeling secure, protected, safe, and serene. (Pause.)

Feel the love, the caring, and the concern radiating from this being inside you. (Pause.)

Feel yourself relax into it more and more, further and further, now. It is so good. (Pause.)

The radiance passes over your entire body. The warmth and love envelop and cradle you. (Pause.)

Answer it! Say to yourself: "Yes, I feel the peace, the security, the love. I feel whole and complete just as I am at this moment. This moment is perfect." Rest in this moment. (Pause.)

Know that you can return to this place of serenity any time you wish, any time you are silent and still, open and accepting. Simply be silent and expectant, but not forceful in your inward listening. Be expectant as if you are about to hear the most important message in the world. You will hear it, for it is. Once you touch this inner being, allow it to converse with you. You will discover that life can be a celebration, and you're invited. Come just as you are!

Now, it is time for you to return to the room around you, to this experiencing. Begin to awaken yourself by gently stretching. Think again: "My body is relaxed and my mind is peaceful." Complete this thought with: "I am whole and complete, just as I am at this moment. This moment is perfect." Stretch fully with an energizing yawn, and a grateful smile to take with you.

Have you ever really SEEN the starry night?
Or, did you just "look" at the distant constellations?
Shanti — Shanti — Shanti — Peace — Peace — Peace

ADVANCED LEVEL 1 LESSON 10

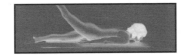

I commend those of you who have reached this lesson. We never really stop growing. We must keep learning in order to grow; we must keep doing to grow. If you decide to take a break from your lessons at this point, remember the following basic principles:

- Watch what you eat. If you continually eat highly seasoned foods your body/mind cannot reach the calm state that is needed for meditation.

- Watch what you drink. Stimulants of any kind—alcohol as well as coffee, tea, and caffeinated drinks—are disturbing to a calm state of being.

- Watch your morals. You are trying to reach a state of higher consciousness in meditation, and you can't do that with the bad conscience that low morals causes.

- Keep your body in shape so that it will not disturb you with pain or discomfort when you are sitting in meditation.

- Learn to control your breath. If you learn nothing else in yoga class, learn that! It is so essential, not only physically, but mentally. It is the doorway to calmness, to controlling the mind so that you can enter meditation and be more peaceful in life.

- Don't expect, demand, or force the meditation. Just be open, aware, awake to the moment. It will happen, probably when you least expect it.

- Be less bound by your ego. So what if someone spells your name wrong? That's only your I.D. It is not really you. Remember, all your cravings and hurts and wants and unhappiness are of the ego. You are complete, just as you are.

- Try to bring some naturalness back into your life. Don't live in a totally false world of human fabrications twenty-four hours a day. Go back to your naturalness. Naturalness is wholeness, and it's found in nature, outdoors.

- Put simplicity back into your life. Eat, live, play—learn to just be—as uncomplicated as possible. You'll be healthier and happier. Remember your carefree days of youth? Try to recapture them.

- Remember this one well: I want you to laugh right out loud at least once a day. Just laugh. Even a smile changes the whole chemistry of your being. Laughter is such a healing thing. Laugh aloud, at least once a day. Laugh at yourself! That's a great healer.

There are many methods of meditation, and no one method is right for everyone. That's why we do it differently each week. You are a different person each day, so why should you do the same thing every day? It's okay: be different. We all must seek out and discover what is most advantageous for our own particular personality, at our particular level of consciousness. Remember, meditation is not a holy ritual to be performed once or twice a day. It is a method of consistently seeing things clearly, consciously, here and now.

 # Continuities

Now it's time for you to center yourself, relax, and breathe, and begin your postures. Practice the continuities in a flowing motion in the order listed.

Seated/Reclining Continuity

1. Infant Posture and Stretch #17
2. Upper Body Stress Release #88
3. Gate I #69
4 Gate II #70
5. Elimination #9
6. Wheel #112
7. Raised Bow #65
8. Sitting Spinal Twist #12

Reclining Continuity

1. Forward Frog #20
2. Reverse Frog #21
3. Half and Full Bow #44
4. Half and Full Locust #45
5. Full Rolls and Balance #26

Standing Continuity

1. Toes, Flat, Chair, Tree #15
2. Standing Waist Roll #51

3. Windmill #52

4. Lateral Stretch #98

5. Moon Stretch #99

6. Sun Worship/Sun Salutation #64

7. Pulsing #76

8. Standing Relaxation #64

Relaxation/Meditation: OM II

At the end of the Intermediates lessons, we learned about intoning "OM." We learned to feel its vibrations throughout our being. Now, at the end of this session, we will do the same. So, take a few deep, relaxing breaths, follow your exhalation. Close your eyes. (Pause.)

The original source of your being is One. When you think in two, three, four, or more, you miss the point. You miss truth. Learn to accept everything and person around you as an extension of your being, like the singular diamond with its many different facets. Be open and empty to, willing and waiting in this moment. Think nothing, yet be aware to the experience of all-that-is.

There is the soft silence, the comforting calm, the precious peace, and there is this: love! Feel that love. When you inhale, feel the love fill you. When you exhale, send love outward, again. Fill every corner, every space of this room with love. From floor to ceiling, just love! Warm, comforting love. Absorb it and let it absorb you. (Pause.)

Let us make that oneness verbal with a few rounds of the OM, the One. Inhale and let me hear it, let it vibrate in you and through you. (Pause.)

Now that our oneness has been joined with the One, lie back and cover yourself with the blanket of love that you created. Remember, love is your true nature. You are the result of the love of thousands. Now just rest. (Pause.)

Many times I have said to you that when you live in love you never have to fear. Fear tries to make itself logical to you, and gives you all kinds of reasons for its existence. Love gives you this moment—whole and complete and safe—just as it is. Every moment of your life you are offered the opportunity to choose love or fear; to tread the earth or to soar through the heavens. Choice is a wonderful thing when we use it properly, consciously, knowingly. Trust your heart to show you the way. Your heart is far wiser than your ego thinks it is. The heart is ruled by that inner being that watches over you from the center of your being.

Remember to be centered in your stance as well so that you will feel planted, strong. Feel centeredness in your back and you will feel weightlessness. Feel centered in your head and it will direct you. Keep centered in your seeing and you will know flawless receptivity. Learn to be centered in the sound for it is the silent presence. This is what brings wholeness to your world; being centered and balanced to life. Lastly, learn to stay in the now.

Namaste: when you are within that place within you, and I am in that place within me, we are one! (Pause.)

Gently, ever so gently, take a deep inhalation. Fill yourself with that wonderful, loving prana energy. Bring yourself back to this room, this moment, this now.

Stretch a little, then longer. Really stretch and wriggle your body into aliveness. Take that wonderful, awakening yawn, and remind yourself, "My body is relaxed, my mind is peaceful. I am One with the universe." Smile and laugh!

Every decision you make is an opportunity to grow—to realize your full potential.
All decision comes from our own choosing—make your choices well.
Choose to connect with your inner self—there is no more rewarding experience.
It is returning home—at last. It is pure JOY!
Shanti—Shanti—Shanti—Peace—Peace—Peace

Advanced Level 2 Lessons

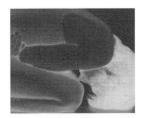

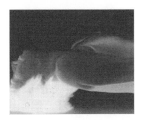

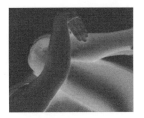

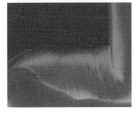

ADVANCED LEVEL 2 LESSON 1

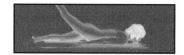

In aerobics class or other types of exercise classes, everyone is expected to perform the same exercise, the same number of times, equally vigorously, regardless of whether or not your body is able to perform at the same level of expertise as everyone else's. When you come to a yoga class, you're treated as an individual because each body is different. If you have been loyally following this book, you are certainly advanced in your yoga practice, and may want to begin tailoring your practice to your own needs. Maybe you don't want to practice the same routine in a lesson every day of the week, and you want to change something. Here is an outline you can follow in devising your own routine:

- Your routine should encompass a full spectrum of postures. Each session should include:

- A twist posture (to keep the spine supple)

- An inverted posture (to relax and renew the inner organs)

- A tensing and releasing posture (such as the Instant Corpse)

- A balanced position for the nerves (such as the Sun Worship/Salutation, which should be performed twice).

On the days you're feeling lazy, start your routine in a reclining position. On days when you're ready to go and you need to calm down, start in a standing position and work your way down. On another day, start with a seated posture and work your way up. In other words, don't get in a rut, don't let your practice get boring and mechanical. Every day is new, and so is each moment and each experience of the postures you do.

For the maximum benefit, try to hold each position at least 30 seconds. Some days you may want to stay in the head stand for only a minute; other days you might want to do it for five minutes. Do not hold any posture if you are uncomfortable in it.

Try to do your postures each and every day. Yoga is one habit that is good for your body. It needs to be stretched and awakened. Your body will perform much better for you if you treat it that way. At the same time, your mind needs to rest. You need to sit and just breathe. The postures become a lot easier and you will be more relaxed, have more energy, and you will certainly live longer. Take time to relax when you have finished your practice. Store that energy that you have created through the movement of the postures. Always think positively: "I *can* do it. I *can* do it."

Some of our postures are fun, and if you feel like laughing at yourself lying on the floor and wiggling like a sleeping puppy when you do Dreaming Dog, then laugh! Laughter is a healer. I've always believed that you can be sincere without being serious. So, if we laugh it's not because we are not serious about what we do. We are very serious. But laughter makes it so much better.

Doing postures early in the morning sets the pace for the day. By stretching the body awake, by starting the circulation moving we move more freely through the day. We have more energy. After your postures, it's best if you can just sit for a moment or two—five, ten, fifteen minutes—to just sit and breathe, and bring yourself into your inner self. Give yourself a positive thought that your day will be good and that nothing will interfere with your calmness during that day. When it's time to go to work or to whatever you have to do during the day, you will be better prepared for it, and the day will move better for you.

Now, we'll start by reminding ourselves how to breathe. Sit with your eyes closed, try to keep your back fairly straight, ears above shoulders, nose above navel. Your back is straight but not stiff. Inhale very deeply, and your stomach pushes out. You want to fill yourself with energy, that wonderful prana energy, that oxygen. When you exhale, pull your stomach in. You will be doing this for a few moments to relax yourself, to get the stress out of your body, empty yourself of all extraneous thought. Then, your body will be ready to do the postures. After the postures, you can lie down relax. Let's breathe.

Continuities

The first week of a new session is always devoted to a review of postures we have already had. There are no new postures. Remember that the continuities present the opportunity to achieve a continual flow of movement. You learn to become the posture instead of simply doing one posture, stopping, and then doing another posture. By becoming the posture, your body automatically flows from one posture into the next, into the next, and so on. With no break in the movement or the flow, your practice becomes a meditation.

Reclining Continuity

1. Dreaming Dog #1
2. Lie and Stretch #2
3. Leg Raise I and II #3
4 Reverse Bow I and II #4
5. Lying Knee to Head #31
6. Upper and Lower Rolls #43
7. Head to Knee and Pull #6

Seated Continuity

1. Butterfly and Advanced #19
2. Sitting Backward Stretch #36

3. Sitting Leg Stretch #27

4. Anterior Stretch #39

5. Sitting Spinal Twist #12

6. Kneeling Reverse Arm Raise #10

Standing Continuity

1. Standing Backward Stretch #50

2. Standing Head to Knee #13

3. Knee to Elbow Lift #46

4. Standing Wall-Ceiling #30

5. Sun Worship/Sun Salutation #64

6. Swim Down #94

7. Jonathan Balance #73

8. Sun Relax #62

Relaxation/Meditation: Leaf Visualization

The body likes movement, especially the gentle, flowing movement of yoga. It feels energized and, at the same time, it is calmed and relaxed, centered, and balanced. In movement, the mind is removed from the humdrum requirements of getting through the day, and it also becomes calm, quiet, and peaceful. Now, let's see if we can deepen that peacefulness and learn to just be.

Let's try to become one with nature, with the naturalness and oneness of all universality. Set your mind free to soar with the birds, float with the clouds, to be the leaf drifting down to earth, to be the lotus opening up to behold the sun, to be the tree reaching in mutual adoration to the heavens. Learn to become that which you already are!

How do you do this? How do you become the bird, the cloud, a single raindrop? How do you feel as the tree feels? Through the breath! It is the breath that allows you empty the mind, to put aside all the restrictions and limitations of ego that says to you, "Stay here, pay attention to me!"

Why does ego try to control us like this? When we are floating freely among the clouds, when we learn to set ourselves free, the ego becomes smaller and it loses control. The more we practice setting ego aside, the smaller and more insignificant it becomes. So, let's prepare ourselves for this trip.

Lie down gently and quietly on the floor, arms at your sides, body comfortable. Check to see if you have done that properly. Start by asking yourself, "Do I feel comfortable? Is there any part of my body that needs adjusting?" If so, make that adjustment now. Is your lower back comfortable? If not, you might need to slightly raise your knees to correct this. Are your neck and shoulders relaxed? Give them a little wriggle and see. Is the back of your head on the floor or, is your head tipped backward? Adjust it now.

Take one long, slow inhalation, feeling your abdomen push upward. Then, slowly exhale, feel the abdomen return to its natural position. Another long inhalation and the abdomen pushes upward, automatically. This time, as you exhale, feel any remaining tension or stress gently float away on the breath—

out, out, out. Let it all go. Inhale gently and feel peacefulness and calmness enter your being, flowing through your whole body, flowing through your mind, softly calming, quieting. Exhale slowly. Feel your mind becoming more peaceful as you breathe away all thoughts. Feel it become empty. Feel it become still. Continue to breathe gently and slowly. Each inhalation and exhalation leaves you feeling quieter, more peaceful. (Pause.)

Picture a door in front of you. It can be any kind of door you wish, any size, any color. Bring your attention to the door. See it slowly swing open for you and invite you to walk through. Go ahead, walk through. There is a beautiful tree in front of you, any kind of tree you like. See how it glows in the sunlight. It is alive with the joy of being. Walk toward it. Reach out and touch the trunk. Feel its aliveness! Look up at the branches and the leaves. See how the leaves flutter to and fro in the breeze. Pick a leaf. Any one will do. Feel yourself float upward so that you are sitting next to that leaf. Reach out and touch it. What do you feel? Do you feel its life, its joy? How it moves to the wind? Up and down, this side and that side. Do you feel how it lifts itself to the sun? Feel the wind caressing you as it caresses the leaf, and the glow of warmth as the sun touches it. Where does your touch end and the leaf begin? Are you the leaf? Is there any difference? Do you feel as the leaf feels—have you become the leaf? (Pause.)

Meditation is emptying the mind, becoming as all things. It is not subject and object—the leaf and you. Meditation is subject and object becoming one, you and the leaf becoming one.

Everything is the same. In Oneness there is no separation, no dualism; there is only being. When we attach a name to something, we create a separation, and in doing so, we get further away from Oneness. We forget how to simply just be: as the leaf; as the snowflake; as the wind; the clouds; the raindrop. We forget that we and the oneness are One. (Pause.)

On your next exhalation, gently let go of the leaf. Feel yourself float down to the ground. Take one last look at the tree. Feel how it reaches out to enfold you with love. Go back through the door. Turn your head and watch it slowly swing shut. Know that it is never truly closed. It is waiting for you swing it open again any time you wish, any time you are ready to walk through. You simply have to empty your mind, be open to it, and it will open for you. Take a deep inhalation and bring your attention back to your body, to this room, to this doorway to life, to being. Gently stretch. Wiggle your arms and legs. Feel energy flowing back into your body. Give a yawn back to awareness, and remind yourself, "My body is relaxed, my mind is peaceful." Feel it! Be it! Feel yourself smile with the joy flowing through you.

Take time to hear what the winds have to say
The message of the murmuring of water
The beauty of the bird's song
And you will find the truth of life.
You will find joy!
Shanti—Shanti—Shanti—Peace—Peace—Peace

ADVANCED LEVEL 2 LESSON 2

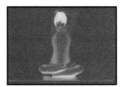

The only failure in yoga is not trying. As much as doing postures and breathing is important, it's important to pause. Most of us get up in the morning, feeling light, relaxed, calm, and quiet. We go to bed at night feeling frazzled, tired, worried, and worn out. Why is this? During the course of the day, we forgot to pause. Of all the things in nature—and that includes us, whether we think so or not—humans are the only beings that have forgotten how to pause. Trees always sway; then, they become still; likewise, the shrub, the flower, the blade of grass. A dog stretches out and pauses. The cat sleeps on the windowsill. The bird rests on the limb. Even the ant takes a break. Not us—we are caught up in the whirl of the world. We create our own problems and confusion.

So, what about the pause? A true pause means a silencing of all mental activity, not just being quiet. Each silence has its own rhythm. There is the silence of the empty building, the silence of an empty house, the silence of an empty church, the silence of the woods, or just the inner silence. So we can be still, as in unmoving; we can have quiet, or we can be silent. Proper silence is a form of meditation. Meditation is controlling the mind; emptying it. Only an empty mind can realize truth. So let us stop, and realize.

The essence of yoga is to help us see life with a new perspective. The eyes see only color and form, but we put names to things. Yoga teaches us to really *see* everything unlabeled. Our ears hear only sound and vibrations As soon as we attach a name to what we hear, we distort it. By naming or labeling, we don't see the reality of it.

Beneficial Hearing

There are three types of hearing: shotgun, basket, and digestive. Shotgun hearing occurs when we hear something in one ear and shoot it right out the other, and retain nothing at all. Basket hearing is when we take something in but the real substance leaks out, leaving only the residue. Digestive hearing is the most beneficial of the three. It allows us to remove all rubbish and absorb what is substantive. Through digestive hearing, you can learn to hear, to see, to smell, to touch, to feel. It awakens your senses. This awakening is also part of yoga, part of saying: "I'm really living. Life is a celebration."

Continuities

Begin your breathing, to relax the mind, the body, to rid it of stress, of thoughts and all hindrances to our enjoyable yoga practice. Just close your eyes and breathe. When you're ready, practice the postures in the following continuities in the order listed.

Seated/Reclining Continuity

1. Fingers (Raindrops) #100
2. Neck Roll #7
3. Turtle #93
4 Shoulder Lift and Roll #8
5. Lotus Relaxed Posture #57
6. Rowing #53
7. Sitting Twist Swing #54
8. Sitting Mill #55
9. Side Scissors #68
10. Side Scissors Variation #102
11. Swan #22
12. Floating Swan #23
13. Balance on Fours #24
14. Cat Variations #28

Standing Continuity

1. Wood Chop #14
2. Bear Walk and Lower #47
3. Sun Worship/Sun Salutation #64
4. Tree Balance #95

New Postures

113. Yoga Triceps Stretch.

This posture can be done either standing or sitting, preferably sitting. Raise your right arm straight up so that the upper part of your arm is next to your ear. Bend your elbow and let the lower part of your arm drop back behind your right shoulder. Reach over your head with your left arm and grasp your right elbow. Gently pull your right elbow behind your head. Refrain from bending your spine, which creates tension in your neck. Try to hold this posture for at least 30 seconds. Repeat for your left side.

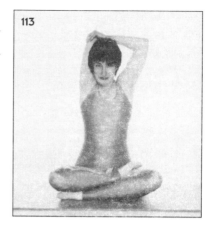

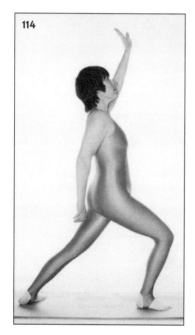

114. Lunge Coordination Walk.

This is similar to the Lunge Stride (#105) with a few exceptions. Instead of raising both arms above your head when you lunge forward, raise the arm that is opposite to the foot forward. For example, if your right foot is forward, then raise your left arm is raised, and vice versa.

115. Frog Lift Variation.

This posture is a variation of Raised Frog (#83). However, in this variation, in the kneeling position, your hands are placed on the outside of your knees. Your body is first raised halfway, and then all the way.

Relaxation/Meditation: Body Awareness

Some people consider their bodies as their whole being and feel that without the body, there would be no being. In fact, the body is so important to some of us that we sometimes are overattentive to it and exercise excessively. Still, with all this effort toward the body, we truly know very little about it. We often forget to listen to it, to heed it, and, more importantly, to experience it. In this relaxation, we are going to use intense concentration to experience our body more fully. This intense concentration is also a preparatory state for entering into meditation.

Begin by relaxing on the floor. Close your eyes and center yourself. Take a deep inhalation that allows you to enjoy the thorough exhalation of letting your body go loose and limp, released and relaxed. (Pause.)

Did you really note how your body felt when it made contact with the floor? Did you feel the weight of it let go? Did you notice if your body rested on the floor completely, from head to heel, including the back of your legs, your buttocks, your back, your shoulders, your arms, and your hands? Did you really feel your body, or did you move it unconsciously? If so, you missed the experiencing of it. Unfortunately, this often occurs to many of us. The following exercise will teach you to concentrate more thoroughly, to experience more thoroughly, by going over your entire body.

Begin at the top. Very slowly, simply open and close your eyelids a few times, and notice how they feel more relaxed each time. Continue opening and closing your eyelids, until you really don't want to open them again. Move your jaw around, and let your lips relax into a tiny smile. Did you feel the muscles of your cheeks relax? If you'd like, you can yawn and feel even greater movement. At the end of your yawn, rest your tongue near the roof of your mouth, just behind your upper teeth. Sometimes it's even helpful to frown or wrinkle your face, your nose, your forehead. Then, smile again as your facial muscles relax. (Pause.)

Roll your head gently from side to side. Make sure that your neck muscles are not tense. Feel all those muscles. Although we don't generally pay any attention to muscles, they that can trigger our stress and tension. We often think of these muscles as small and unimportant, but every muscle affects another muscle in the entire network of muscles. (Pause.)

As you inhale deeply, move right and down your body. Truly feel your chest muscles rise and fall. (Pause.)

Continue moving down your body to the area of your abdomen. Contract your abdomen muscles. Feel the movement and the release. (Pause.)

Repeat this movement with your buttocks: Contract them and release them. Experience the movement. (Pause.)

Contract and release your thighs and calves. Experience them. (Pause.)

Repeat this contraction with your feet. Tighten them and release them. Experience the movement in your feet. (Pause.)

Squeeze your fists tightly and feel the muscles in your hands and in your arms. On your exhalation, let everything go limp. Experience the whole procedure. (Pause.)

You should now have a new understanding and appreciation of your body. Keep concentrating on it and relaxed it much more fully. You should learn to concentrate on it, even when you're not doing anything at all. For example, right now, take a fairly deep inhalation and, in the pause between the inhalation and exhalation, experience your own heartbeat. After the exhalation, experience the peacefulness of it. The awareness to the moment and the happening in that moment are very peaceful. (Pause.)

This rest and release, this true peace, should feel good. This lesson shows us that we can control our body. It all begins with thought. This is why it is important to pay attention to our thoughts. If we think negatively, our body feels it and reacts to it. However, if we think positively, our body follows that thought, and then we are in control of our lifeline to health and happiness. Take some time now to simply rest. (Pause.)

Tomorrow morning when you awaken, truly stretch to life! Feel the air fill your lungs. Really see the morning sun, and hear the morning bird in its bath. Feel the slippers on your feet, and taste that morning morsel. Smell the morning breeze. Truly awake and be aware of life, your life. You owe it to yourself! Now, stretch yourself awake in this moment with a positive thought: "My body is relaxed and my mind is peaceful. I am whole and complete just as I am at this moment, and this moment is perfect." Stretch. Yawn and smile.

True seeing is not done with the eyes, but with the soul.
It is not merely an outward vision, it is an inward Knowing.
Shanti—Shanti—Shanti—Peace—Peace—Peace

ADVANCED LEVEL 2 LESSON 3

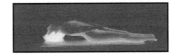

It is very easy to follow the yoga discipline when you are in a class setting. The real accomplishment is in bringing yoga into your everyday life, not just for the hour or so of your practice. Every single one of your movements says what you are, where you are, and who you are. Whether you are walking, running, eating, or brushing your teeth, learn to do so and move gracefully, smoothly, effortlessly, and freely. Learn to stand and sit centered. Always be aware and awake to the potential of your being. This means following the naturalness of being, just as animals do.

The Example of Animals

If you've forgotten how animals move and how they are watch the bear. It always moves from its center. Watch the fox because it teaches us alertness. The wolf teaches us tirelessness. The deer teaches us sensitivity. Flamingos teach us how to step. Crows show us the art of observation. Cats teach us attentiveness without tension. Dogs teach undying love. Animals simply do, without defining their own qualities. They are natural and spontaneous. Let us learn this naturalness, this spontaneous movement to life. The more natural we become to our being, the more free and joyful we'll feel. You might ask: "Should we go to bed when the birds do and rise with the cock's crow?" Maybe. Certainly, we should walk in the rain and warm ourselves in the sun. We should run to the top of a hill and laugh loudly. We should always remember who and what we really are and act accordingly.

Continuities

Center yourself. Begin with your feet—your base, your foundation, your root to the earth. Move up to your heart, where there should be peace, joy, and stillness. Your head should feel a sense of direction. Your mind controls your body. When you see, truly see. Don't simply look at. When you hear, listen to the silence. Now, find your own center. Close your eyes and breathe deeply. Empty yourself of stress and thoughts, and enter into this moment. When you are ready, practice the postures in the continuities in the order listed.

Reclining/Seated Continuity

1. Infant Posture and Stretch #17
2. Upper Body Stress Release #88
3. Lion #3
4. Gate I #69
5. Gate II #70
6. Elimination #9
7. Camel #29
8. Raised Bow #65
9. Forearm-Wrist Stretch #61
10. Half and Full Bow #44
11. Half and Full Locust #45

Standing Continuity

1. Toes, Flat, Chair, Tree #158
2. Standing Elbows to Knee #77
3. Centered Triangle #74
4. Sun Worship/Sun Salutation #64
5. Lateral Stretch #9
6. Moon Stretch #99
7. Circle Earth/Gather Clouds #109

 ## New Postures

116. Holding the Balloon.

Take a stance with your feet comfortably apart, at about shoulder width. Bend your knees slightly, as though you were sitting on a high stool. Raise your arms to shoulder height and form a large circle. Your wrists should be leveled with your shoulders and your elbows slightly lower. Imagine that a balloon supports your elbows. Imagine also that small balloons are under your armpits and one between your thighs. Your weight should be shifted slightly forward, but not out of balance. Do not raise your heels. This is a calming and centering posture. Hold it for as long as you are comfortable.

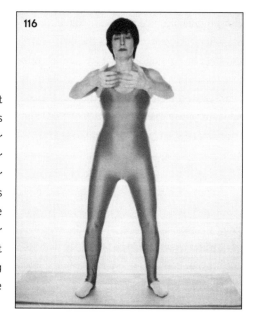

117. Upper Hip Roll.

Lie flat on the floor and raise your knees to your chest. Wrap your arms around your knees as though you were giving them a big hug. Keeping your shoulders and upper back flat on the floor, roll your hips first to the right side and then to the left side. This posture is beneficial to your waist and increases your lower back flexibility.

118. Head Turn and Bend to Side.

Sit or kneel on the floor with your back and neck straight but not tense. First, inhale and gently turn your head as far to the right as you can, as though you were trying to look over your right shoulder. Exhale and return your head to center. Inhale and repeat for your left side. Second, slowly relax your head down to your right shoulder as though you have just dozed off. Slowly raise your head to center, and then relax it over your left shoulder. You are facing forward during this second variation. These postures help to relieve tension in the neck. If you have neck problems, please practice these movements very gently.

Relaxation/Meditation: Complete Relaxation III

This relaxation is a helpful if you've had a very exhausting day, both physically and mentally. You will free yourself of all your stress. It is time for you to take charge of your life, your feelings, and your well-being. Give yourself this positive thought: "This is my time to relax and to really let go." Then, sigh yourself down. Let out a healthy out breath, and allow your body to hear the sigh that tells it to let go. Don't hold back. Don't cheat yourself. You need this pause, this peace, this precious time.

As you let go, picture yourself sinking into a gigantic, fluffy, soft feather bed. Let it billow up about you and cradle you gently and lovingly. Your body sinks down, but you feel light and suspended. (Pause.)

It is acceptable to have a certain amount of rush in your life. But along with the rush, you should relax, revive, renew, restore, and rest. Become placid, peaceful, pleased, and pleasurable by turning off all thinking, all troubles, and all tensions. It means that you should be still, silent, and serene. It means that you should just be! To just be is to experience now and only now at this moment. Being in a state of now-ness is being witness to your is-ness. Sometimes this is called such-ness—the true essence of you. In this state, you can experience without discrimination, without judgment, without attachment. It is total freedom! It is simplicity at its finest. It is witnessing life in its most uncomplicated, unsoiled, untainted form. Everything is as it is! It's not wishing or wanting for anything. It is feeling complete just as you are, where you are, and that you are. Do you feel this? Open to it and allow it. (Pause.)

Absorb the stillness around you, and listen to the silence within you. Let it all be a wordless observation, a peaceful experiencing. (Pause.)

Rest in the moment and let no outside thoughts enter your mind. This is your time. Stay in this time, this experiencing, this allowing. Bask in it fully, and follow your breath. (Pause.)

Where are you now? Are you resting in your repose, basking blissfully? Is your inner consciousness lifting you to new heights of relaxation? Are you drifting in and out, and letting go further and further into that state of peace where the essence of you comes alive? It is right there, right now. Release yourself to it, and let go! (Pause.)

Believe in it and in yourself. That wordless, indescribable calm and content exists at this moment, deep within you. It is always there awaiting your presence, your attention to it, your allowing of it. Allow it now. (Pause.)

Follow your feelings. Trust in you. Trust the being inside of you that has always watched over you, guided you, protected you, and loved you. That is your other self—your true Self—the who and what you are when you pause long enough to experience it. When ego is laid aside, the being of you comes to life. Learn to recognize you and learn to know you! Take the time now to rest for a moment, still sunk deeply into that soft, billowy, fluffy feather bed that is cradling you ever so gently. (Pause.)

Take a deep inhalation, and, as you exhale, let out a loud sigh, a giant: "Aaaaaah." Begin to stretch, gently at first. Once again reinforce your positive thought: "My body is relaxed and my mind is peaceful. I feel whole and complete just as I am at this moment, and this moment is perfect." Stretch fully stretch, yawn, and smile. Surely, if you meant what you just said to yourself, you do feel like smiling. Life is a celebration, and you are invited. Come as you are.

Take time each day to nurture yourself.
It's the best way to say thank you to God for your life.
Take time to serve others.
It's a debt owed. Repay it!
Take time to laugh.
It's music to God's ears!
Shanti—Shanti—Shanti—Peace—Peace—Peace

ADVANCED LEVEL 2 LESSON 4

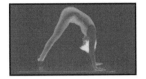

Discomforts such as headaches, colds, and backaches are all too common. In spite of aspirin and other drugs, people still get headaches. Drugs simply suppress the pain, but the cause of the pain is left untouched. Pain is a warning to the body.

Headaches: Causes and Cures

Suppressing pain can mean that its cause goes unheeded and, therefore, can become worse. The most common causes of headaches are tension, poor elimination, and poor diet. Tension can be reduced through proper breathing, and elimination can be improved with the Elimination posture. Diet can also affect headaches by causing obesity, which results in extra stress on your spinal column. Alcohol expands the blood vessels in the body and brain. We are all familiar with the effects of caffeine.

Headaches can also be caused by overexposure to the sun, poor ventilation, overly tight clothing, dehydration, smoking, and vision problems. What can you do to eliminate these problems? You should begin by regulating your exercise, your food, and your breathing.

Once you've identified the cause of your headaches, many natural therapies and remedies are available. These include: pressure point therapy, chiropractic treatment, homeopathic remedies, hot foot baths (to draw the pressure and congestion from your head), and body detoxification. You can also try to improve your diet by eating more fruits and vegetables, drinking pure water, taking food supplements—particularly vitamins A, C, E and calcium—and drinking herbal teas. Conventional headache products only promise relief. They do not address and cure the cause. When you relieve pain, you suppress it; you don't cure the cause. The problem may become worse and develop into something more serious. So listen to your body when it talks to you about pain!

If you truly follow the yoga way—move your body, breathe properly, eat properly, practice relaxation/meditation—you probably won't get a headache. If you do get a headache, try practicing the Neck Roll, the Shoulder Lift and Roll, or simply sit and breathe. You should try to help your body naturally. Try not to harm it with drugs. You can be your own best healer, if you listen to your body.

Continuities

Listen to your breathing. Close your eyes and release all stress and thoughts, even your headache if you have one. As always, practice the postures in the following continuities in the order listed.

Standing Continuity

1. Standing Backward Stretch #50
2. Tension Mill #92
3. Back and Hips Rotations #96
4 Standing Hip Strengthener #71
5. Wall-Ceiling Variation #85
6. Toe Toucher's Squat #72
7. Sun Worship/Sun Salutation #64
8. Pulsing #76
9. Sun Relax #62

Reclining/Seated Continuity

1. Fish #5
2. Lying Knees to Floor #35
3. Plow and Variations #40
4. Pelvic Lift #41
5. Three-Quarter Shoulder Stand #42
6. Full Rolls and Balance #26
7. Shoulder Lift and Roll #8
8. Neck Roll #7
9. Fingers (Raindrops) #100

New Postures

119. Snake.

This posture is an uninterrupted Swan (#22). Instead of stopping or resting between each separate movement of the Swan posture, simply keep moving into each part of the posture in one continuous, flowing movement. Keep moving through the positions for as long as you are comfortable. Lie on your stomach with your hands on the floor under your shoulders. Inhaling, lift your body straight up. Bend your knees and raise your buttocks up. Moving backward, slide your hands along the floor and relax back onto you heels. Your forehead should be close to the floor. To come out of this position, push your hands forward along the floor. Your nose also moves along the floor. Your buttocks rise up into the air, and your body follows your hands forward. At the full extension, inhale and lift your body up to the Cobra position. Exhale and move backward again. Your arms are outstretched and your forehead is close to the floor.

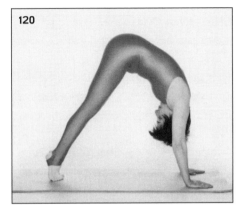

120. Stretching Dog.

Kneel down with your hands flat on the floor in front of you, but do not sit on your buttocks. Inhale and raise your body so that you are supported by your hands and toes. Your head should be between your arms. Your body will look like an inverted V. Exhale and lower yourself down to your knees.

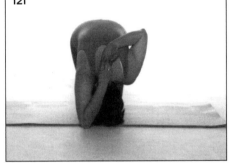

121. Head of the Cow.

Kneel down on the floor, but do not sit on your buttocks. Inhale and raise your right arm up and over your right shoulder. Your fingers are behind your shoulder. At the same time, bring your left arm behind your back. The back of your hand is against your back. Interlock the fingers of both hands behind your back. Exhale and bend forward to place your head on the floor. Inhale to bring your body up and release your arms. Inhale and repeat for the opposite side of your body.

Relaxation/Meditation: Active and Passive Concentration

In this session, begin by practicing sitting for a few minutes. You'll try your concentration on what is known as active and passive concentration. Adjust yourself comfortably in your sitting position with your back straight, but not stiff, ears over your shoulders, nose above your navel, and eyes closed. Take a few deep, relaxing breaths, if you wish. Let your breath be smooth, flowing, almost effortless. (Pause.)

Begin with the active form of concentration. In this form, you are concentrating on your breath and excluding all else. You'll allow no other thoughts. Count one as you inhale and exhale; then count two as you inhale and exhale, and so on. Try to reach the number ten without any outside thoughts. If a thought occurs, start over again at one. Simply keep breathing from one to ten. You may begin now. (Pause for three to five minutes.)

In the passive form of concentration, you sit and breathe calmly and relax thoroughly. You can let your mind drift wherever it wants to go. In this form, thoughts will occur. The trick is not to hold on to them. As quickly as they form, let them fade away. Do not become involved or attached to your thoughts. If you try to hold on to them, become involved or attached, more and more thoughts will arrive. Thoughts never seem to travel alone! The best way to practice this is to see each thought as a bubble. Watch it rise up, drift away, or just burst. Do whatever works for you. Give it a try. (Pause again for three to five minutes.)

Keeping your eyes closed, gently and slowly lie down, centering yourself comfortably on the floor. Allow a relaxing breath as you let your body go loose and limp, released and relaxed. (Pause.)

Continue with the counting system of relaxation. This time establish in your mind that the number ten is very special. It is a relaxing number. (Pause.)

Hold this thought in the positive section of your mind. Inhale, exhale, count one and think relax. Again, inhale, exhale, count two and think relax. Keep doing this exercise until you reach the number ten. Knowing with absolute certainty within yourself that when you reach ten, you will be totally relaxed. Begin now. (Pause for three to five minutes.)

You are now totally relaxed physically and mentally. Accept this present moment as a precious gift and fill yourself with it. Stillness and pause, calm and serenity, utter peacefulness now envelop your body and mind. It is what you have longed for, what you needed the most. It is a form of salvation to your inner and outer being. There is no safer, more placid plateau of existence, and it is yours now! Realize it and fill yourself with it and bring it back with you. In a moment, you will start to count backward from ten to one, knowing that when you reach one you will awaken fully and feel totally rested and revived. Begin your count back. Inhale, exhale, and count ten. Inhale, exhale, and count nine. Continue to number one. (Pause three to five minutes.)

You are back, rested, and revived. Enjoy this for a few moments and dwell within it, storing this feeling to take with you when it's time to go.

A mindful, working, and successful practice takes positive thinking. It takes trusting yourself. It takes faith and a quiet knowing inside of you. These qualities take time to acquire and you may not feel quite as rewarded this time as you will in future practice. However, you should still feel rested and more peaceful. No practice is ever wasted. Each time you try, you are that much closer to success and to your state of bliss, the bliss that you so deserve.

You should not so much focus on the quantity of time you spend practicing, but on the quality of your practice. Those who try the hardest will generally get the most out of their practice. If the practice seems a little difficult for you right now, be of good cheer, because you will probably reap the greatest reward. Reward yourself now with a gentle stretch and your positive thought: "My body is relaxed and my mind is peaceful. This moment is perfect." Enjoy a full stretch, a joyous yawn, and a wonderful smile.

We Awaken when we finally realize
that all our thoughts are just thoughts.
Our Joy is experiencing the reality
that follows our dissolved thoughts.
Shanti—Shanti—Shanti—Peace—Peace—Peace

ADVANCED LEVEL 2 LESSON 5

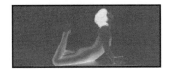

Conventional medicine does not cure the common cold. At best, it relieves it. We think colds come from being close to someone who sneezes, or from a draft, a germ or virus. Actually, colds come from a condition called toxemia. *Tox* stands for the toxin or poison and *emia* means blood. Just as *anemia* means poor blood, *tox*emia means poisonous blood. We can get toxemia through the intake of poisonous or spoiled foods and through the body's inability to quickly eliminate the waste and toxins accumulated by overeating or eating the unhealthy foods. Negative thinking, which is most detrimental, can also trigger toxemia. For example, if you walk into a room and somebody repeatedly asks if you are alright and tells you that you don't look too good, then you might begin to feel as though there is something wrong with you. The opposite is also true. Assume that you don't feel well, and someone says to you: "Gosh, you really look wonderful!" Wouldn't you immediately begin to feel better? It's all in a thought, a thought that someone else can place before you, or one that you can decide on for yourself. Positive thinking has a lot to do with feeling well, so practice it for yourself. Try not to rely on others to do it for you.

Curing the Common Cold

Toxins in the bloodstreams can be discharged in three ways: through the kidneys and urinary tract, through the pores and sweat glands, and through the mucous membranes.

You can sweat out toxins with physical labor or exercise, performed every day. Working up a good sweat every day increases your longevity.

It is most important to encourage mucous discharge. Try not to suppress it with antihistamines that stop your runny nose. When you stop your nose from running, your cold will last longer because you retain the mucous in your system. Why would you want to hold this in your body? Let it run, and get it out of your body.

Fever is another friend of the cold. It sweats it out of your system. When you have a cold, try to stay away from pastry, starches, and animal fats. These foods slow down the digestive and elimination process, thus keeping toxins in the body longer. You'll notice that most colds occur right after a holiday, when we eat excessively. In fact, fasting can be one of the best treatments for a cold. Your fast doesn't have to be long or overly strict. Begin by consuming only liquids, soups, juices, and water. It will flush out your system quickly, and you will feel lighter and healthier.

Our bloodstream becomes overloaded when mucous producing foods—such as milk, cheese, cream, butter, eggs, red meat, white bread, and starchy foods—are consumed in excess. Try to eliminate or at least cut down on these types of foods, and you will have less mucous in your system, and, therefore, fewer colds.

Another effective remedy for a cold is to take some extra vitamin C and garlic when you feel a cold coming on. Try not to wait until you have a full-blown cold before taking these remedies.

Many herbs can also treat colds. Always read the recommended dosages on the label, and remember that more is not necessarily better. Certain acupressure points can relieve the discomfort that comes with having a cold. You can learn the acupressure points that apply to your particular discomfort and become your own healer.

Continuities

Breathe deeply and release all stress and outside thoughts. Then relax into your postures. Close your eyes and breathe. As always, practice continuities in the order listed.

Reclining Continuity

1. Dreaming Dog #1
2. Lie and Stretch #2
3. Leg Raise I and II #3
4 Reverse Bow I and II #4
5. Ceiling Walk and Cross #34
6. Ceiling Walk Variation #101
7. Half Bridge #103
8. Head to Knee and Pull #6

Seated Continuity

1. Butterfly and Advanced #19
2. Anterior Stretch #39
3. Sitting Leg Stretch #27
4. Sitting Spinal Twist #12

Standing Continuity

1. Grasped Fingers Behind Back #80
2. Temple Fingers Behind Back #81
3. Crossed Arm—Front and Lower #82
4. Sun Worship/Sun Salutation #64
5. Lunge Stride #105
6. Skater #49

New Postures

122. Modified Cobra.

Lie face down on the floor as in the beginning of Cobra posture (#16, position 1). Inhale and raise the upper part of your body as in Cobra. At the same time, bend your knees and try to touch the back of your head with your toes. Exhale to lower your body down. This posture is quite difficult for most people. Only move as far as it is comfortable for you, and don't try to force your body.

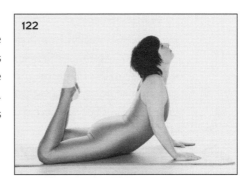

123. Extended Toe Squat.

Take a standing position with your heels together and your toes comfortably facing out and to the sides. Turn out from your hips, but do not twist your knees or ankles to turn your toes further to the side. Inhale and raise your arms straight out in front of you. At the same time, rise up on your toes. Exhale and lower your body down into a squatting position, balancing yourself on your toes. Stay in this position for as long as it is comfortable. Inhale to raise your body, while staying on your toes. Exhale and lower your arms, and drop down onto the flat of your feet. This posture strengthens your legs.

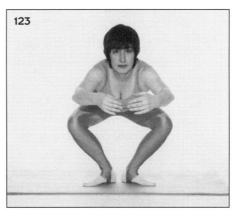

124. Tension Twist.

Lie on the floor on your back with your knees bent and the flat of your feet on the floor. Raise your arms up and onto the floor behind your head. Twist the upper part of your body from side to side. Keep your buttocks on the floor and twist only from the waist up.

Relaxation/Meditation: Shift Breathing

We practice shift breathing when we become aware of the shift from inhalation to exhalation and from exhalation to inhalation. Adjust your body comfortably with your back straight, but not stiff, your ears over your shoulders, and your nose above your navel. Rest your hands on your lap or along your thighs, and close your eyes. You will not participate actively in the shift from one breath to the other, rather, you will simply witness the subtleness of it, the smoothness of it, or the unevenness of it. Remember that you should not try to control it. Simply be aware of your breath. Follow the rhythm of it, allowing it its own course. This practice is to teach you concentration and to stay in the moment, to be with what is happening. If you are open to it without any restraints, the following of the breath will calm and relax you. Begin now. (Pause for three to five minutes.)

Keeping your eyes closed, slowly lie down and adjust your body to the floor, centered in comfort, released and relaxed. Feel your muscles become loose and limp, as you take a full exhalation that lets you settle down and in. Having followed the shifting of your breath, you should already feel physically and mentally relaxed to the moment.

With your body at ease, concentrate on your mind. First, select a color. Choose a calming color: blue, green, aqua, or lavender blue. Don't choose an energetic color, such as orange, red, or yellow. When you have your calming color, picture it as a glowing ball of light shining right above you, not brilliantly bright, but soft, subtle in its glow. Picture it now. (Pause.)

Try to truly experience the presence of your light-color, not only with your inner viewing, but with feeling. Feel it as a warm glow, a soothing, loving glow that shines down upon you in a gentle stream of light. (Pause.)

Let this gentle stream of light grow in size and watch it fall upon your entire body like a gentle mist—a sheer blanket of mist touching you warmly and covering you from head to toe. Feel it especially on the exposed parts of your body. It caresses your face and your hands with warm, comforting light. It is relaxing and also refreshing. Simply enjoy it. (Pause.)

Begin to feel this warm, comforting light wrapping itself around you. Experience its soothing touch, not only in front of you, but beneath you. Feel enveloped in a cocoon of light, suspended and equally as light—free! Feel it. (Pause.)

Where does the light end and where do you begin? You can no longer distinguish. You are one, and it is good! This moment is truly perfect. Rest in it. (Pause.)

You will now begin to let these gentle streams of light recede upward again, very slowly withdrawing upward from your sight, but not from your feeling. Concentrate on keeping the same feeling of being enveloped and cocooned. (Pause.)

Your body is soothed and relaxed, and your mind feels peaceful. You feel the hint of a smile upon your lips as you think to yourself: "Yes, this moment is perfect!" And now, there is just a very dim, distant glow far above you. Let it, too, fade as you rest for a moment. (Pause.)

When you come back to the room around you and to your wakefulness, again, ask yourself who is waking. Recognize how you are wakening. Is it in a state of serenity, calmness, and restfulness? Do you feel revived and at peace? When we are open and accepting of the moment, of the happening, and engaged in the experiencing, we are all of these things and a little more that is always indescribable. When we touch the infinite, finite words can't describe it. That is how it should be.

Remember this as you begin your half stretch to wakefulness and as you repeat your positive affirmation: "My body is relaxed and my mind is peaceful. I am whole and complete just as I am at this moment, and this moment is perfect!" Fully stretch, yawn, and smile!

What is the easiest thing to do?
What is the hardest thing to do?
The answer to both is: BE HERE NOW!
Be present in the moment. TOTALLY present!
Shanti—Shanti—Shanti—Peace—Peace—Peace

ADVANCED LEVEL 2 LESSON 6

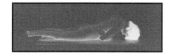

Over fifteen million Americans suffer from arthritis. Ninety-seven percent of all individuals over the age of 60 develop some form of arthritis. Based on these numbers, there is a fairly good chance that you might get arthritis, unless you do something to prevent it. Let me preface this by saying that there is no reason that you should get arthritis; there is no need to, if you follow your yoga practice. Arthritis is a dichotomy: It can be due to a loss of calcium in the joints, and it can be caused by a build-up of calcium. It is an imbalance between calcium and phosphorous in your body.

Relieving Arthritis

Rheumatoid arthritis is the most common form of arthritis. It attacks the fingers, toes, elbows, knees, and other joints through loss or lack of calcium. Therefore, this form of arthritis needs calcium. I'd like to point out once again that sugar, caffeine, and alcohol seriously disturb the calcium/phosphorous balance in your body. If you consume these products, you may also need to take additional phosphorous to balance your intake of calcium. But it would be best to avoid these products completely.

It is also helpful to eliminate all processed foods, including breads, cakes, fast foods, meats (including chicken), packaged foods (including parboiled or partially cooked packaged rice), dairy products, fats, oils, fried foods, and carbonated drinks. You might be wondering what there is left for you to eat. Try basing your diet on fresh raw or steamed vegetables and fruits. If you feel that this is not enough, gradually add almonds, which are rich in oil and protein, and whole steamed grains. You can also drink raw juices, such as carrot, beet, parsley, alfalfa, wheat grass, and even potato juice. However, fruit juices should be used sparingly. The healthiest juices are fresh, not processed, sour apple and pineapple. Whenever possible, eat only vegetables and fruits that are in season in the area where you live. In the winter, if you live in a northern climate, you should try to eat more root vegetables and bitter greens, and less fruit. If you live in a southern climate, you are lucky enough to have fresh fruit available year round.

I have known people who have had terrible arthritis problems. Some of these people, who were almost completely bedridden, changed their diets to only vegetable and fruits, and, after a couple of weeks, noticed wonderful changes in their bodies. Sometimes, however, as soon as people begin to feel better, they believe that they are cured and return to their old eating habits. Invariably, their arthritis returns. If you continue to eat a diet of fresh foods, your body will thank you for it. Remember, you are not born with arthritis. You develop it through your habits. Furthermore, just as you created the ailment, you can also remove it from your system.

When you activate your body, you also relax your brain. Any movement of the body is calming to the mind. Therefore, practicing your postures is a form of meditation.

 # Continuities

Sit for a moment, and then begin your movement. When you are comfortable, take a few deep breaths and empty yourself of stress and outward thoughts. Bring your awareness to the now. Close your eyes. When you are ready, practice the following continuities in the order listed.

Seated Continuity

1. Fingers (Raindrops) #100
2. Head Turn and Bend to Side #118
3. Neck Roll #7
4. Turtle #93
5. Shoulder Lift and Roll #8
6. Sitting Backward Stretch #36
7. Lotus Relaxed Posture #5
8. Reverse Balance Leg Lift #104

Reclining Continuity

1. The Cobras #16
2. Modified Cobra #122
3. Infant Posture and Stretch #17
4. Reverse Frog #21

Standing Continuity

1. Skeleton #18
2. Airplane #37
3. Standing Twist #38
4. Sun Worship/Sun Salutation #64
5. Jonathan Balance #73
6. Standing Relaxation #79

New Postures

125. Triangle Variations.

First Variation: Stand with your feet well apart, with your hands on your hips. Inhale and raise your right arm over your head and turn your palm to face the left. Turn your left leg outward so that your toes point to the left side. Do not twist your knee. Exhale and bend your left knee, and lower your body down to the left side. Your right palm will be facing the floor, and your right leg will be extended. You'll want to give your right leg a good stretch. Inhale to raise your body. Exhale to return your right arm to your hip. Repeat for the left side of your body.

Second Variation: Assume the same stance as in the first variation—feet apart and hands on hips. Inhale and raise your right arm and turn out your left leg. Exhale, bend your left knee, and slide your left hand down your thigh to your bent knee. Your right arm stays vertical pointing to the ceiling. In this position your torso is more upright that in the first variation; there is not as much stretch to the right side, and you do not bend your body over your left leg. Inhale to raise your body. Exhale to return your right arm to your hip. Repeat for the left side of your body.

126. Standing Gravity Alignment.

Stand in a centered position with your feet below your hips and your knees relaxed. Drop your head and chin down to your chest. Let your shoulders droop and your arms hang loosely. Exhale, as you very slowly begin to bend your body forward. Gradually, your body folds in half until your hands rest on the floor in front of you. Simply pause there. When you are ready, inhale and slowly begin to roll (not lift) your body up.

127. Crocodile.

Lie face down on the floor with your legs shoulder width apart. Allow your heels to fall inward. Bring your arms in front of your head and fold them at the elbows, placing your right hand on your left

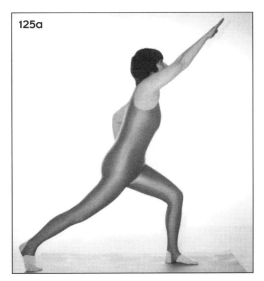

125a

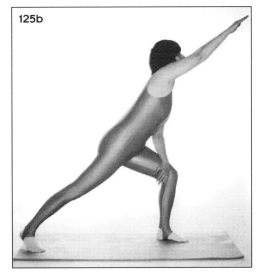

125b

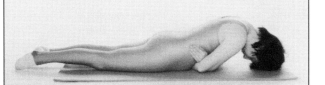

127

elbow and your left hand on your right elbow. Draw your arms closer to your body and rest your forehead on your arms. As you do this, your shoulders and rib cage should lift off the floor. Close your eyes and breath deeply and evenly. Hold this posture for as long as you are comfortable. This pose is very good for the solar plexus, for balancing, and for easing fatigue.

Relaxation/Meditation: Earthing

Our moods and our needs change. We change. Your way of reaching peace is unique to your own needs. By learning a variety of so-called ways to meditate, you will hopefully find at least one form that is successful for you. However, you should try to always remember that the doorway to all of these methods is the control of the breath; there is no passage, no entering the true state without it. All openings to meditation are made accessible by the breath.

Sit comfortably erect with your eyes closed. In this exercise, we will use sound. Choose your own personal mantra. The most popular is OM. You may wish to simply use OH or AH. A one-syllable mantra is the easiest way to begin. Your sound should be prolonged; rise from your abdominal area—the center of your being—pass through your throat area; and come out at your lip or tongue area. It should carry the full vibration through each area so that you feel it throughout your body. Your sound does not have to be loud. It can be a very quiet personal sound, but it should be strong enough for you to feel the vibration through your whole body. Begin chanting.

(Chant for three, four, or five minutes.)

While keeping your eyes closed, slowly lower yourself to the floor. Center your body comfortably, and relax your breath. Release a final, full exhalation. The form of relaxation you will now learn is known as earthing. It is a way of getting back in touch with nature, a state that we should never have left.

Instead of seeing yourself and feeling yourself resting here on this floor, in this room, picture, instead, that you are outdoors, stretched out on a soft plot of grass on the side of a small hill. Simply sink into the grass. It will feel good. Let go. You are alone, but you are not lonely. It's a beautiful day! Just right! The sun is warm upon your face and hands. It's not too hot. It is a comfortable warmth. You feel a gentle breeze pass over you. Can you feel it? It feels good. (Pause.)

Two things are happening. Try to experience them. If you remain open to this experience, you will feel a new nurturing take place within your body. When you inhale feel the warmth of the sun, not only on your outer self but inside you. It fills you with energy as well as warmth. Every time you exhale let yourself go a little further. Sink down a little further as if your outer body were melting into a oneness with the soil beneath you. It is a gentle blending, a joining, an experience of oneness. Try it now. (Pause.)

Keep breathing in this energy, this nourishing and nurturing energy source from deep within the earth. It is the same source of life-giving energy that is generously given to each plant, each tree, and each flower that blooms. Feel yourself intimately joined with this earth energy, as you exhale and release yourself to this source. Become a true part of the ecological group called earth. Revisit your source to life. (Pause.)

When we merge to oneness, we re-emerge to our wholeness. Feel whole now. Cherish the nurturing that you have just received. Feel new, revived, and refreshed. Feel a wellspring of new life burst inside you. This experience is not only a physical change, it is a mental and spiritual change as well. It calms your mind and inspires your spirit. All great beings found their higher understanding and aspirations by going out into the wilderness. We all have the same potential for greatness. Nurture yourself with a last full inhalation and bring it back with you to this now. Gently stretch back to aliveness. As always, add your affirmation: "My body is relaxed, and my mind is peaceful. I am whole and complete just as I am at this moment, and this moment is perfect!" Fully stretch and yawn peacefully, and smile. You are home!

When you finally see God in ALL things,
you will be connected with your true source.
WELCOME HOME!
Shanti — Shanti — Shanti — Peace — Peace — Peace

ADVANCED LEVEL 2 LESSON 7

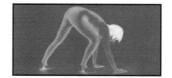

There are indications that one of the main causes of cancer is lack of oxygen in the cells. This fact alone should prompt you to practice yoga and deep breathing regularly. Without food and oxygen, normal cells evolve abnormally into neoplastic cells. Consequently, cancer develops from these cells. Why do cells lack oxygen? The number one reason is from lack of exercise. *Move*. Get your heart pumping to help in the exchange of fresh air. Stress and emotional and psychological factors also cause blood vessels to constrict, thus interfering with the flow of blood and the transfer of oxygen to the cells. Other known causes of cancer are chemical food additives and environmental conditions, such as poisoned water and polluted air.

Cancer: The Diet Connection

A poor diet is a major factor in cancer development, particularly an excessive protein consumption from meat, eggs, cheese, and other dairy products. If you consume more protein than your body can process, the excess becomes a waste product in your system; it becomes ammonia. Ammonia interferes with, and slows down, the growth of normal cells, and speeds up the growth of cancer cells. We need red blood cells to be healthy. Leukemia, for instance, is an overproduction of white cells. It is interesting to note that white cells always increase after meat consumption. People who eat diets very low in fats and without meat have very low incidences of cancer.

It's also interesting to note that thousands of cattle and chickens have shown to have cancerous disorders. This, of course, is not surprising when we take into consideration all the chemical additives, antibiotics, and growth hormones that are pumped into these poor animals. Unavoidably, by consuming meat, we also consume the chemicals that are injected into these animals. The chemical additives, specifically the nitrites and nitrates used in ham, bacon, corned beef, hot dogs, and sausages, result in toxins in our liver. As these chemicals clog our liver, they prevent it from cleansing our blood. This increases not only our chances of developing cancer, but other diseases as well.

The best cancer prevention is to stop consuming cooked, devitalized, and processed foods. Try to switch to a diet of live foods, such as fresh, raw vegetables, fruits, juices, whole grains, and seeds.

Supplement your diet with minerals and vitamins, and exercise regularly. A fast is a good detoxifier for the body. You might want to educate yourself on the numerous benefits of specific vitamins and supplements. It is your body, and you should learn to take care of it. Nature created a perfect world. The things that interfere with this wonderful, natural world are man-made. Nature intended for us to enjoy good health. It is up to us to eliminate our bad habits and to decide that we really want to live and be healthy. The choice is always ours.

Continuities

Choose to breathe. Choose to bring your inner awareness awake. Cast out all stress, all frustrations, all thoughts of the day. Simply relax, and close your eyes. When you are ready, practice the continuities in the order listed.

Seated/Reclining Continuity

1. Infant Posture and Stretch #17
2. Upper Body Stress Release #88
3. Lion #11
4. Gate I #69
5. Gate II #70
6. Elimination #9
7. Camel #29
8. Raised Bow #65
9. Hinge #60
10. Swan #22
11. Floating Swan #23
12. Balance on Fours #24
13. Cat Variations #2

Standing Continuity

1. Standing Head to Knee #13
2. Standing Waist Roll #51
3. Windmill #52
4. Sun Worship/Sun Salutation #64
5. Circle Earth/Gather Clouds #109

New Postures

128. Great Physical Breath of Yoga.

Proper attention to each movement and to each inhalation and exhalation will allow you to feel the energy flowing from your palms to your head, heart, stomach, and spine. Your concentration should be held on each position for at least 30 seconds. Stand with your feet comfortably apart and your arms at your sides. Inhale and raise your arms. Interlace your fingers over your head with your palms facing downward. Raise your arms upward with your fingers still interlaced. Feel the energy flowing down to your head. Exhale and release your fingers, and allow your arms to fall to shoulder height at your sides. Bring your arms to the front and interlace your fingers. Inhale and bring your hands to your heart area. Concentrate and feel the energy from your palms to your heart. Exhale and release your fingers. Let your arms fall to your sides, then to the front at stomach level, and interlace your fingers. Inhale and bring your palms to your stomach. Feel the energy flowing into this area. Turn your palms to face the floor. Exhale and push downward, still concentrating on your stomach area. Inhale and raise your arms to waist height. Exhale and release your fingers. Bring your arms behind your lower back and interlace your fingers, with your palms facing your spine. Inhale and bring your palms to rest on your lower back. Feel the energy flow into your back. Turn your palms to face the floor. Exhale and push downward, still concentrating on your lower back area. Inhale and raise your arms up to waist height. Exhale, release your fingers, and let your arms fall slowly to your sides.

129. Spine Strengthening Exercise.

This position is fun and easy! Just ask your dog or cat. Walk on all fours around the room. You can either move your right hand and right foot at the same time or alternate between the two. Try it both ways. This posture strengthens your upper back and adds flexibility to your hip area.

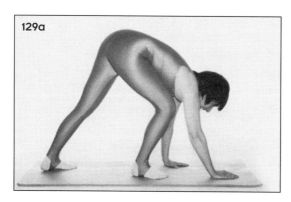

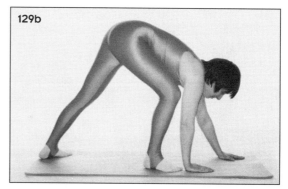

130. Stretch/Open Eyes/Yawn.

This pose is a good release after doing a lot of sitting postures. It is also another very easy posture! In a sitting position, reach upward with your arms, as high as you can, and stretch. Open your eyes wide and squeeze them shut, then open wide again. Yawn big—nice and wide. Let out a big sigh as you yawn, maybe an "Aaaaaah." This posture helps you relax before continuing with other postures.

Relaxation/Meditation: Walking Meditation

Because it is sometimes difficult for Westerners to sit for long periods of time, many yoga classes allow a reclining position. In more formal training, as in Japan, meditation is mostly practiced in a sitting position. In most temples, the sitting period lasts for at least forty-five minutes; meditation then continues by walking. Many students find that this method works well for them. You should remind yourself that whenever you try something different for the first time, it will not become truly relaxing until you are accustomed to it and make it a part of yourself. For example, although you were probably excited the first time you learned to drive a car, chances are that it wasn't a very relaxing experience. You might have been too nervous and unsure of yourself. Unfortunately, some of us are too relaxed when we drive. Our mind is elsewhere, anywhere but on the driving. We become so comfortable that we forget to pay attention.

In a walking meditation, you should never become so relaxed that your mind is not on it completely, with it completely, and absorbed in it completely. If you are not paying attention, you will miss the point and the rewards of it.

Begin by moving to one side of the room. Stand comfortably centered. Be sure that your feet are below your hips, and feel yourself firmly planted. Your knees are slightly relaxed. Your back is straight, but not stiff, and your shoulders are relaxed. Tilt your head, slightly forward. Almost close your eyes, and gaze about three feet in front of you at a spot on the floor. Your breathing is relaxed and coming from the center of your being, around your navel area. (Pause.)

Your pace should be slow, much slower than you have ever walked in your entire life. The more slowly you move, the more beneficial this will be. When this exercise in practiced in yoga classes, some teachers believe that walking meditation is best done with the students in a circle, in order to show that no one wins and no one loses. I agree with this belief for very advanced classes, where the students are accustomed to walking meditation and are fully aware of the energy connection to each other. However, in classes where students are new to this type of meditation, I feel that it is better to walk in a straight line so that each student can develop his or her own rate of travel to the opposite wall.

Place the back of your left hand in the palm of your right hand, with both palms facing up, and hold them in a relaxed manner close to your body, about waist high. Your pace will be slow, but not so slow that you begin to wobble and fall off balance. Until you become accustomed to this practice, give yourself these reminders: "Shift, lift, place, move." You should practice this until the movement becomes automatic. *Shift* means that you are shifting your weight to one side of the body. *Lift* means that your are lifting your opposite foot, the foot with no weight. *Place* means that you should lower your raised foot, heel first. *Move* means that you should transfer your weight to the original balance of 50 percent weight in each leg. In order to continue, simply begin the process by shifting your weight to your front leg, then continue. Make each step deliberate, but don't plop yourself down. The placing of the foot should be gentle and soundless. Move with confidence, with dignity, and feel regal. Your steps should be very short, no greater than half the length of your foot. Try to remind yourself that this is not a race, but an awareness. Truly feel each shift, lift, place, and move. Practice this for at least ten minutes.

Keep thinking: shift, lift, place, move. Move from your center, and make sure you do not slouch. Move with dignity, assuredness, and total awareness of the movement. (Pause.)

Your body reflects dignity, grace, effortlessness, smoothness, and peacefulness. Let that be your whole being. (Pause.)

Try not to force your movement or you might become tense. Simply remain balanced and centered. Move from your middle, from hara or dan tien—your center between heaven and earth. (Pause.)

Pause for a moment, and feel the calm and the peace of your being. Take this peace with you as you slowly lie down, still centered in your being, and exhale a sigh of relaxation. For the next few minutes, you may choose any surrounding you wish. It could be a soft plot of grass on a hill, a sandy beach, or an area in the woods. Simply choose whatever atmosphere is most pleasing to you at this time. You can even stay within your walk, and imagine yourself moving slowly about the room. Simply relax, without hurries, hassles, or wants for anything. Feel complete and content, just as you are at this moment. Know that this is the perfect time to just be. Let everything else wait because this is your time. (Pause.)

When you are ready, leave your surroundings and come back to the room around you, to this now, this experiencing. Stretch softly to wakefulness and affirm: "My body is relaxed and my mind is peaceful. I am whole and complete just as I am at this moment. And this moment is perfect." Fully stretch, yawn, sigh, and smile. You are home.

A little thought?
There are no "little" thoughts, only many parts of a larger thought.
Is a pebble insignificant?
Watch the effect the ripples make.
Shanti—Shanti—Shanti—Peace—Peace—Peace

ADVANCED LEVEL 2 LESSON 8

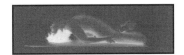

We need a certain amount of stress in our life or we wouldn't have any life at all. However, prolonged, out-of-control stress becomes *dis*-stress. One is a positive type of stress, while the other is negative. Positive stress contributes to life, while the other contributes to disease.

Lowering Blood Pressure with Yoga

Medical doctors have studied the effects of yoga on blood pressure and anxiety. After six weeks, almost all of the sixty-two people tested, showed a five to ten point decrease in their blood pressure level. These tests, as well as many others, revealed that proper yoga breathing, for thirty seconds, reduced blood pressure for thirty minutes. If we breathed properly all day, we'd be in pretty good shape.

Additional medical tests also concluded that yoga proved most effective in reducing stress levels. Three specific techniques were suggested for maximum benefits: Hatha Yoga, various relaxing methods, and meditation. The study concluded that our bodies need movement and that these particular methods help us reduce stress and enable us to cope better in our daily lives by fully using our bodies. Most people do not perform strenuous physical work every day. Fortunately, Hatha Yoga moves the body, fully but gently.

In our practice of yoga, we develop our concentration and become aware of the changes we must make in order to lead healthier lives. Yoga helps us become more aware of our inner being. As we become more centered and more balanced, we become calmer beings. With regular yoga practice, our entire existence becomes more flexible—physically and mentally. Consequently, if our minds are flexible, we are able to release and relax and better deal with any stressful situations. As we continually remember these practices, we bring ourselves into a closer harmony with nature. Our meditation shouldn't be only an occasional practice. We should become it. Meditation creates the ability to look at things as they are. It allows us to face our problems calmly, as they are. It teaches us how not to turn molehills into mountains. Meditation calms and balances our body. A calm and balanced being flows through daily life easily, with the flow of life itself.

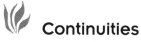

Continuities

Breathe quietly, and rid yourself of stress and outer thoughts. Turn inward. Simply close your eyes and breathe. When you're relaxed, practice the following continuities in the order listed.

Standing Continuity

1. Standing Backward Stretch #50
2. Tension Mill #92
3. Back and Hips Rotations #96
4 Standing Hip Strengthener #71
5. Wall-Ceiling Variation #85
6. Toe Toucher's Squat #72
7. Sun Worship/Sun Salutation #64
8. Wall Twist #89
9. Side Wall Twist #90
10. Half Moon #91

Reclining/Seated Continuity

1. Fish #5
2. Tension Twist #124
3. Leg Up/Sit Up #63
4. Forward Boat #33
5. Infant—Palms Down Stretch #107
6. Infant—Arms Up Back Stretch #108
7. Forward Swing Breath #66
8. Hare #32

New Postures

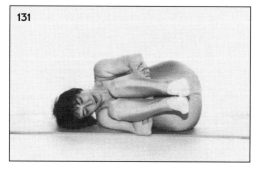

131. Round Rolls.

Sit on the floor with your knees bent and your hands clasped underneath your knees. Roll back until your back is on the floor and your clasped knees are upward. Roll around on your back in full circles: on one side of your back; on your lower back; on the other side of your back; and, finally, on your upper back. Rotate in one direction, then stop and rotate in the opposite direction. Stay relaxed. This posture loosens up and massages your whole back.

132. Advanced Fish—Lotus.

Lie on your back. Bend your knees; place your legs in Lotus position (#57). Keep your arms at your sides. You may hold your feet with your hands if you wish. Raise your upper body and place the top of your head on the floor. Your buttocks stay on the floor. Be sure that your weight is on your elbows and not on your head or neck.

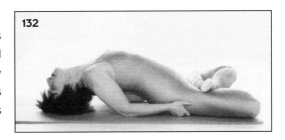

133. Standing One Leg Stretch.

Stand with your feet about one foot apart. Inhale, bend your left knee, and raise your left leg. Hold your left foot with your left hand and stretch your leg and arm forward. Exhale, release your foot, lower your leg. Repeat for your right leg.

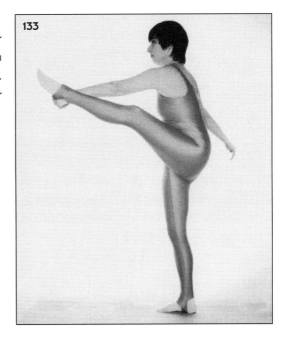

Relaxation/Meditation: Kneeling Meditation

Kneeling meditation combines movement, from the waist up, and nonmovement, from the waist down. If you are not used to kneeling, or if you have bad knees, you may be more comfortable with a small pillow or your rolled-up mat placed under your buttocks, which will raise your torso slightly and keep pressure off your knees. This style of meditation is called Zen sitting, and it can be quite comfortable with practice, even more comfortable than Full Lotus sitting style traditional in yoga.

When you are settled, take a few deep, relaxing breaths and close your eyes. Choose an inspirational image on which to direct your concentration, perhaps an image of Jesus, Buddha, Kwan Yin, the Mother of Compassion, the Virgin Mary, a saint, or the Universal Force. Take your time, for this is with whom you will be communicating.

Once you have chosen your image, simply sit for a moment and picture the individual clearly. Hold the image in your mind and in your heart. (Pause.)

Keeping your back fairly straight and relaxed, but not stiff, inhale and stretch your arms up and out. Drop your head back slightly as though you were looking up at the person you have selected. Picture this person in your mind. Bring your arms together, cupping your palms upward as though you are gathering something. Exhale and bring your arms down toward your heart center.

Pause briefly and fill yourself with whatever you have brought back. Then, repeat this movement over and over again. Inhale as you reach up. Pause, and gather in. Exhale and bring your hands back to your heart. Pause again before repeating the movement.

Whatever or whoever you have chosen to gather, meet it as an embrace, a longing, a wanting, a desiring. Be sincere in your reaching, your enfolding, and your gathering to you. Reach with gratefulness and appreciation. Fill yourself. (Pause.)

Be receptive and open to the filling and to the feeling. Let it flow into you, over you, and all around you. (Pause.)

You are showing your gratefulness and your humility, and, thereby, demonstrating your greatness. It is by being humble that we rise to greater heights. Each time you practice this meditation, you will find a fuller peace. Feel it now. (Pause.)

Do you see that radiating image? Is it smiling at you? Is your heart smiling at this moment? That is the feeling you want to absorb and fill yourself with. This time, when you bring your hands back to your heart center, hold them in a prayerful pose for a moment, then lower your head down to them. Pause for a few seconds, then release your hands out to your sides and down.

Gently and slowly, while keeping your eyes closed, lower yourself down onto the floor. Feel relaxed, centered, and comfortable. You are empty and filled at the same time. Cover yourself with this feeling of love. Your heart is full from the communication that you just experienced. Rest.

It is through meditation that we are able to glimpse into the blessedness of the Infinite, the Everlasting, the Pure and Holy, the untarnished reality of *Is*-ness. You should never be afraid to take the gigantic leap from finite to infinite experiencing, from prisoner to prince or princess, from fatuity to freedom, from pain to peace, from bewilderment to bliss!

Realize how you feel right now, at this moment. Have you ever felt more content, protected, watched over, and loved? You can feel this way anytime you wish by being silent and going within. Treat yourself to this pause that refreshes, renews, reaffirms, redirects, and reassures us of who and what we truly are. We are precious and perfect, as we are. There is nothing for us to become. We must only realize our self. Did you realize? If you did not realize this time, you will when you are ready.

Prepare yourself to come back to the room around you and to this moment. Gently stretch back to aliveness. Affirm to yourself: "My body is relaxed and my mind is peaceful. I am whole and complete just as I am at this moment, and this moment is complete." Learn to say this to yourself. Stretch fully, yawn, and smile from the joy in your being.

Take the time to ask: What is the purpose of my life?
Then be very quiet so you can hear your heart's answer.
Shanti — Shanti — Shanti — Peace — Peace — Peace

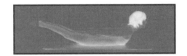

Most foods that we buy in the supermarket have lost all of their nutrient value through being harvested unripe and through long shipping and holding periods in cold storage. Food, particularly fruit, that is picked before it has a chance to fully mature, cannot have developed the equivalent nutrients as fruit that is picked at the peak of its growth and placed immediately on the plate. There is no fresher food than that which you grow yourself.

Vitamins and Minerals

Some of us may feel that a once-a-day vitamin covers all our vitamin and mineral needs. However, once-a-day vitamins are geared for the "average body." Vitamins have more value when taken individually because specific vitamins are more likely to suit your body. Water-soluble vitamins, such as vitamin B and C, are very important. Since they are water soluble, we can't overdose on them, and any excess is washed out of our system. Brewer's yeast, for instance, is a complete, balanced vitamin B in natural proportion to the other B vitamins. In other words, it does not contain 50 mgs or 100 mgs of all the B vitamins. Most research shows that brewer's yeast has twelve to fourteen individual B vitamins. If you don't like the taste of brewer's yeast, then consider primary, grown yeast. This comes in powder form and, when mixed with liquids for a drink, tastes nutty. Vitamin B keeps us from becoming tired, irritable, nervous, and depressed. It also helps with constipation and insomnia.

Vitamin C comes in two forms: Natural C, which contains all the citrus bioflavonoids, and Synthetic C, which is ascorbic acid. Both types are beneficial to your body, and will keep you free from colds. Vitamin C interacts with other vitamins to aid in healing and is also excellent for fighting infections.

Vitamins A, D, E, and K are oil-soluble, which means that they remain stored in your system for varying periods of time and should be taken in low dosages. As with all vitamins, always follow the directions on the bottle. Vitamins A is an antioxidant and wonderful for the eyes and skin; it helps your immune system and aids in the prevention of cancer. Vitamin D, as you all know, is called the sunshine vitamin. It increases the body's absorption of calcium and phosphorous, protects against muscular weakness, and helps build and strengthen bones. As we get older, we need more vitamin D, but only in recommended dosages. Vitamin E has recently gained prominence in treating heart disease because of its benefits to the circulatory system. It is an antioxidant and strengthens the immune system. Although vitamin K is often ignored, it is very important in helping the blood to clot.

We should make sure not to overlook minerals, which are found in kelp and alfalfa. Vitamins control our body's appropriation of minerals, but, in the absence of minerals, vitamins have no function. If our system is deficient in vitamins, it can still make use of minerals; but if we lack minerals, any intake of vitamins becomes useless.

 # Continuities

Think inwardly, and pause. Breath very deeply in and out, in and out. Empty yourself of today's stress and thoughts. Just relax, and close your eyes. When you are ready to begin, practice the continuities in the order listed.

Reclining Continuity

1. Dreaming Dog #1
2. Lie and Stretch #2
3. Leg Raise I and II #3
4. Reverse Bow I and II #4
5. Upper and Lower Rolls #43
6. Lying Scissors #59
7. Sit-up Twist #84
8. Rowing #53
9. Sitting Twist Swing #54
10. Sitting Mill #55

Standing Continuity

1. Kiss the Foot #25
2. Standing Wall-Ceiling #30
3. Wood Chop #14
4. Bear Walk and Lower #47
5. Sun Worship/Sun Salutation #64
6. Temple II #87
7. Temple I #86
8. Holding the Balloon #116

New Postures

134. Easy Cobra.

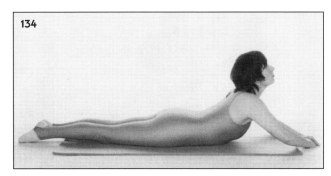

This easier variation is for those who might have difficulty with other Cobra postures (#16 and #122). Lie face down on the floor with your hands under your shoulders. Bend your elbows, slide your arms forward, and clasp your hands in front of your head. Slowly slide your arms toward your body and rest your forehead on your clasped hands. Inhale, slowly raise your head, and look toward the ceiling. If you are able, as you raise your head, try to raise your upper torso off the floor. Exhale to lower your body and head. Even though this is an easier version of Cobra, it still improves your circulation and keeps your spine flexible.

135. Flying Bow.

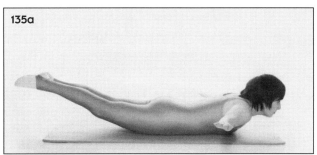

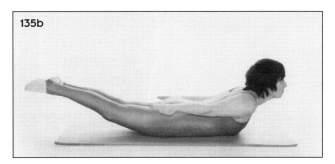

Lie face down on the floor with your arms stretched out in front of you. Your arms and legs are apart. Inhale and lift your arms and legs as in Half Bow (#44). Balancing yourself on your stomach, bring your arms to your sides then, to the back. Return your arms to your sides and again to the front. Your legs remain raised, while your arms move from front to side, to back, to side, and to front, as though you were flying. If you have difficulty going through the full rotation and keeping your legs raised, stop and lower your legs after each arm movement. Simply remember to raise your legs again when you are ready to continue.

136. Pelvic Lift Variation.

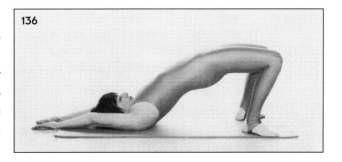

Lie on your back with your arms by your sides. Raise your knees and bring your heels as close to your buttocks as you can, as in Pelvic Lift (#41). Do not hold on to your heels. Inhale, raise your pelvis, and, at the same time, raise your arms up and back, so that they rest on the floor behind your head. Exhale, lower your body, and bring your arms back to your sides.

Relaxation/Meditation: The Path to Oneness

The word "meditation" is a dichotomy: You are alone, yet you are in oneness. You are alone in the sense that you must make the journey and have your adventure alone into that other consciousness. However, meditation is a oneness in the sense that you are not alone when you are in that other state of consciousness. You are one with everything and everyone, with the entire universe! Your oneness is so inclusive that neither the past nor the future exists. All time is right now, right here! You are experiencing everything all at once, with no division, no separateness—a totality! It is fantastic! Wonderful! Breathtaking!

Since we must travel alone, this meditation is designed to help you to enter that state in aloneness, feeling not lonely but complete and content. By now, you probably feel quite comfortable locking the rest of the world out and locking yourself in, putting your ego aside and experiencing your inner self. This meditation emphasizes and teaches you the power that your mind has in creating and disintegrating. It teaches you concentration.

Begin by moving to the wall. Sit facing it, and as close to it as possible. You may sit in either crossed-legged Lotus position (Indian style) or on your heels (Zen style), whichever is most comfortable for you.

Close your eyes and take a few relaxing breaths. (Pause.)

Begin by feeling the presence of the wall in front of you: its massiveness, its solidity, and its permanence. Feel its total presence. (Pause.)

Feel it as a shield against the outside world. (Pause.)

Enforce this image by picturing the wall extending outward, down your right side about as high as your head. Feel it. Experience this extension, as much as you experience the wall in front of you. (Pause.)

Let the wall extend down your left side to the level of your head. This wall is as firm and as solid as the one in front of you and the one on your right side. Truly feel it there, permanent and solid. You feel protected, safe, and comfortable. (Pause.)

Finally, you will close the wall behind you. If you are claustrophobic, don't be concerned because the top is open. Close the wall behind you, again about head high. Feel its presence and the entire solidness of the walls on all four sides of you. (Pause.)

You are all alone, but you do not feel lonely. On the contrary, you are content, safe, secure, and protected in your own little world. Absorb the feeling of this the wall that surrounds you—the aloneness—without fear or panic. It is completely peaceful and so silent that you can hear your breath, the beat of your heart, and the feel of your pulse. Observe it all. Feel it all. Know it all. Experience you in silence and wordlessness. (Pause.)

You can hear the loudness of the silence when you pause long enough to truly listen. It shouts loudly! Listen to it. (Pause.)

Is it not peaceful to rest in your own inner-ness, to experience you minus the ego? Feel it. (Pause.)

Feel this moment, this feeling, this breath, this peace, this wonderful now without thought or analysis. (Pause.)

This is the peace that cannot be seen, touched, tasted, smelled, or heard. But, it can be experienced, felt, and lived. Live it now.

Follow your breath. Simply let it fall from you at will, at its own pace, its own rhythm. Let it fall, and feel that moment of no breath with only the presence of the heartbeat and the pulse in the hands resting in your lap. Open yourself to it. (Pause.)

When you are ready to come back, let the wall disappear once more. Let go of the wall behind you and feel the openness there. (Pause.)

Then, take away the wall from your left side, and let it disappear. (Pause.)

The wall on your right side must go too. (Pause.)

Only the shielding wall in front remains. Release yourself from it now by simply lying back, as if you were stretching out on a soft plot of grass, relaxed and comfortable. Sink in and rest for a moment. (Pause.)

Feel at peace with yourself and at peace with all around you. Be content to just be in the moment. (Pause.)

Your aloneness was not loneliness because you reached the oneness that is ours when we open ourselves to it. We only become lonely when we forget who and what we are. When you realize that you are an important part of the whole, of the One, you will be content and at peace anywhere, at anytime. Most importantly, you will feel truly loved! You have inherited the right of happiness, but you must claim it. You must truly open yourself to it. When you are still and silent, it will appear.

Return to the room around you. Gently stretch yourself back to aliveness, affirming: "My body is relaxed and my mind is peaceful. I am whole and complete just as I am at this moment, and this moment is perfect." Stretch fully to this moment. Yawn and smile. You are home!

Why do you think that you are incomplete when you stand alone in life?
Each being is whole and complete.
Anything or anyone added is extra.
Shanti—Shanti—Shanti—Peace—Peace—Peace

ADVANCED LEVEL 2 LESSON 10

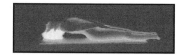

First of all, I want to sincerely congratulate all of you who have made it this far. I'm very proud of you, and, certainly, you should be proud of yourself. I wonder if you feel better, if you feel you've grown, if you're satisfied with yourself. Are you more aware of your body—of your breathing? Are you attuned to your meditation and what it really does for you?

Let your five senses come alive, more aware. Try to really see objects, not just your impression of them; really hear sounds, not what you name them; let the nose experience smell; let your touch have the sensitivity of the things around you; witness your taste. Why? Because experiencing reality teaches us awareness, to stay within this moment, and it gets us out of ourselves and more into the oneness of all else. It is pleasurable, calming, and growing. It helps us back to our naturalness of being. When we begin to experience and realize our oneness with everything there's less need for formal meditation, for the results of this experiencing reality is in and of itself a peaceful, joyful state of being. Again, the most advantageous place to experience reality is outdoors: absorb it, be absorbed by it. Knowledge, or true wisdom, is in the experience of life as it is. It is never authentically obtained from books or even from listening to others. My message to you is learn to use your senses. Learn to have an awareness of now, to be silent, to trust yourself. No one can give you any more than you already have and already are. At best, they can only teach you how to become aware of it. The effect, the reward is totally yours. Remember, your search for the paradise of life will be in your attitude, not in the destination. When you stop looking, you will really see!

 ## Continuities

Remember to practice the postures in the continuities in the order listed, and in a flowing movement from one posture to the next.

Seated Continuity

1. Fingers (Raindrops) #100
2. Head Turn and Bend to Side #118
3. Neck Roll #7
4. Turtle #93
5. Shoulder Lift and Roll #8
6. Sitting Backward Stretch #36
7. Sitting Leg Stretch #27
8. Anterior Stretch #39
9. Forward Frog #20
10. Wheel #112
11. Kneeling Reverse Arm Raise #10
12. Infant Posture and Stretch #17

Standing Continuity

1. Toes, Flat, Chair, Tree #25
2. Knee to Elbow Lift #46
3. Standing Elbows-to-Floor #78
4. Lateral Stretch #98
5. Moon Stretch #99
6. Sun Worship/Sun Salutation #64
7. Lunge Coordination Walk #114
8. Swim Down #94
9. Pulsing #76

Relaxation/Meditation: OM III

And so we come to the end of another growing period. We have learned some new postures, some new relaxation/meditation methods, and, hopefully, we have learned more about who we are, where we are going, where we want to be, and what we wish to become. By now, having touched that inner you in silence, you should be viewing life more positively and joyously.

Adjust yourself comfortably, sitting firmly as a mountain, eyes softly closed, breathing relaxed. Now picture the houses and other living quarters around your own. If you are lucky enough to live in the country or the woods, without a lot of neighbors, then include all the places the animals live in as well as your far-flung neighbors. See in your mind all the beings living around you, doing the different things they do. Connect with them, not analyzing or judging. You are an extension of them. Imagine a golden cord passing from you to each being around you. Through that cord beats one pulse.

The original source of your being is one. Let us make that oneness sing with a few rounds of the one OM. Inhale and let it vibrate in you and through you, going through the golden cord to all around you. When you hear OM, remember what it means: OM is awakening to the Divinity that we are, absolute love, the beingness of total soul. Intone OM until the golden light fills you and then rest quietly. Thank everyone for being alive; thank yourself! Gradually return your awareness to the room and rest.

Change is possible. You only need to change your thought. You have already proven change is possible, for you are certainly different than when you started your lessons! You have learned to unfold and enfold, casting out the old and embracing the new. You're learning to love yourself, you have become more loving and more loveable. The world needs that; it needs the uniqueness of you. You are a very special part of the whole universal plan, one that would be out of balance if there were no you. Every part of you is important, from the breath you send out, to the thoughts you send forth, to your movement upon this earth. Keep that movement centered and balanced; sure footed but light as the wind! Learn to say "Yes!" to now and all the nows, and you will find peace and all that joy you thought was outside yourself. Mindfulness and simplicity in life should be your goal. Then, one day, enlightenment will just happen when you least expect it, but only when you have readied yourself for it. You are nearing your readiness; do not turn back now!

When we enter the moment totally,
God is there to greet us.
Shanti — Shanti — Shanti — Peace — Peace — Peace

Advanced Level 3 Lessons

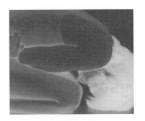

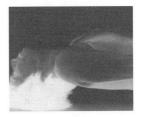

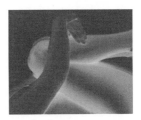

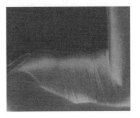

ADVANCED LEVEL 3 LESSON 1

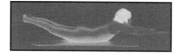

Everyone wants to feel good, to be healthy, to be fully alive. Unfortunately, few of us realize the work involved in attaining that goal. The reality is that only we can do that for ourselves. If we rely on others for our health, on outside influences, on stimulants to make us happy, we rob ourselves of truly knowing total joy. Worse, we become slaves and we become dependent. Yoga is our opportunity to become a totally healthy, happy, complete individual. Yoga helps you to realize all that is already yours. All yoga does is bring it forth, to make you aware of it. You can have what you are seeking, if you only stay with it. You are seeking. If you weren't, you would not have bought this book.

Over these next ten weeks we will be reviewing a lot of the postures that we've already had. We'll be learning a lot of new postures—at least one new one each week—except for this week. We'll be increasing our breathing capacity. We'll be learning new ways to relax and new ways to meditate.

What is your aim, your goal, your desire? Your simplest answer would probably be to be healthy, to be happy. Some of us think we know what that means. Sadly, most of us don't really know. It's nothing like we have imagined it to be or have even been told what it is. A lot of times we have been fooled and misled and we have simply followed the wrong path. We have allowed ourselves to be led by outside influences and by our own ego. But, the ego is really not to blame. It doesn't know as much as our inner self. The ego's capacity for knowing can only go to the extent of its limits. I know that your ego and others have told you that happiness is made up of material wealth, success, fame. I hate to burst the bubble, but it's not for total, lasting completeness. This is not to say that you can't enjoy these things if they come your way. Of course you can enjoy them. But, do not think that the little appetizers of life are the full course. They are the small parts of the feast that awaits you. The lavish, magnificent banquet of life lies before you.

Not too long ago, I was watching television and listening to a man who had AIDS. He was dying. He had all these things that I have just mentioned: material wealth, success, and fame. But, in his final days, what do you think he wished for? Were these things really important to him, what he really wanted, what he really desired? No. What he wanted was to be able to sit outdoors in the park, to smell the breeze, to see the grass, watch the trees waving. Think about it. This was a man, who in his last days, could have anything, *anything* that he wanted, and he chose things that many of us don't even pay attention to, things that many of us don't even desire or love. Nearing the end, he learned that real joy is found in the simple things of life.

Our aim here is to help you to find the same things, before it's too late. It always amazes me how people travel to distant places to witness miracles, when they stand each day, each moment, amid countless miracles. Every leaf that pops out on a tree is a small miracle. Just look around you. Could you have thought of the thousands of different things around you and the intricate workings of each one? How about night turning into day, the sunrise, the seasons, all those stars up there? The delicate spider's web, a fish's gills, the lines in your hand—all are different! Fantastic! And we take it all for granted, even if we notice at all, and so miss life and its simple joys. So our aim, our job, our goal for the next ten weeks is to do our postures with awareness; to breathe properly; to relax totally; and to become more attuned to life around and within us, so we can be truly happy.

With that thought in mind, let us begin. We're going to start by breathing. Inhaling, pushing the stomach out. Exhaling, pulling the stomach in. Keeping your eyes closed to shut out the thoughts of the day, all the stress. Let's just sit and breathe for a moment, and then, we'll do our postures.

Continuities

This first week is devoted to a review of postures we have already had. There are no new postures. With the practice of continuities, you are learning to practice postures in a particular order that allows you to achieve a continual flow of movement. One group may all be performed from a lying or prone position; the next group may be those of a standing position; the third group may be postures in a sitting position. The order of the types of groups (sitting, lying, standing) will change from week to week. In some weeks, depending on the complexity of the new postures and time involved, we may only have two sets of continuities.

Some of the postures we do in continuities are very basic and primarily for beginners. Let me just say that we are all beginners in the sense that we are learning all the time. As you should know by the time you reach this level of study, the purpose of yoga practice is body/mind balance. Even the simplest of postures is beneficial in achieving this goal.

Reclining Continuity

1. Dreaming Dog #1
2. Lie and Stretch #2
3. Leg Raise I and II #3
4. Reverse Bow I and II #4
5. Lying Knees to Floor #35
6. Ceiling Walk and Cross #34
7. Fish #5
8. Head to Knee and Pull #6

Seated Continuity

1. Sitting Spinal Twist #12
2. Elimination #9

3. Reverse Frog #21

4. Stretching Dog #120

5. Hinge #60

6. Hare #32

Standing Continuity

1. Standing Head to Knee #13

2. Warrior #110

3. Triangle Variation #125

4. Sun Worship/Sun Salutation #64

5. Toe Toucher's Squat #72

6. Great Physical Breath of Yoga #128

7. Sun Relax #62

Relaxation/Meditation: The Circle of Life

Now, close your eyes and just sit for a moment. Remind yourself gently that there is nothing more important than just being, right here, right now, totally in the present moment, aware, attentive, accepting. Be fully open to this moment, this experience. Awake and aware, paused and peaceful, content and contained to what is present in this moment. Give yourself permission to be fully open to all that this moment, alive to the now. Keep your breathing relaxed, flowing smoothly, effortlessly, ever so peaceful: in and out, in and out, unforced. Allow it its own rhythm.

Imagine yourself sitting in a huge circle, right in the center. Understand the significance of a circle. In nature, the circle is the law of ultimate growth—the day to day, light to dark, sun to rain, season to season, life to death, to new life again. The cycle goes on, growth goes on, the universe continues.

The planets orbit in a circle. The American Indians' Medicine Wheel is a circle. For the Zen Buddhist, a circle means the opening of enlightenment. The symbol of Taoism is the circle of yin and yang, the perfect balance of harmony in all things. Even our dogs and cats circle about before lying down to peaceful rest.

In a circle, all things are equal; none come before or after the next; none has a better vantage point than the next. All are in the flow, yet with nowhere to go, for each is constantly arriving home in the present moment.

You are an important part of that circle encompassing many individual rivulets merging into the great ocean, or a magnificent diamond with its many facets sparkling as one great light. Know that now, as you sit quietly. For just a few moments, give that circle of great light vibration by humming gently to yourself. When you are filled with that vibration, you may lie down, eyelids closed gently, body relaxed even on the floor, released and relaxed totally.

Always continue to unfold the master within you, take control of your life physically, mentally, emotionally, and spiritually. Have faith in yourself! Changing moment to moment—and letting that change be a new growth, a new understanding, a new completeness of your real self—you are living fully. You can do it! You are limited only by your thoughts, so change them. Start each day with a positive thought, a loving thought. Remind yourself that you are loved, loving, lovable, and see if the day doesn't go better for you.

At times, you might fail and fall into forgetting, but you will also awaken again, and each time you remember, the delight in your heart will explode into a million twinkling stars. But don't wait for this perfection to happen before you start to really enjoy life. Celebrate yourself now for the giant step you have already taken. Applaud yourself, give yourself a party, if you wish. Dance in the streets, kick up your heels, throw your head back and laugh aloud! Don't forget to take a bow. Realize you are not a beggar at the table of life; you are an honored guest! *Namaste.*

> *When you stop naming and labeling things*
> *you'll see them as they truly are; how they are.*
> *It's called reality!*
> *Shanti—Shanti—Shanti—Peace—Peace—Peace*

ADVANCED LEVEL 3 LESSON 2

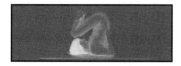

hat is *stillness*? Each day starts with stillness, the stillness of the dawn before the sun rises and before the birds start to sing their joy to the glory of the awakening day. This stillness is the path of meditation. Meditation can be compared to the long stillness before daybreak, when there is nothing but a quietly increasing light. The gradual dawning of a new world is our consciousness, which comes about silently. It is a secret, inner transition that we can never fully share with others. It's a silent path. In other words, the arrival, or the experience of it, simply is. However, the result of our awakening completely alters our relationships with others. We begin to see others differently, and others view us differently. Once we have experienced this different consciousness, we begin to truly see others, whereas before we only looked. This new seeing is a new understanding, a new insight. It is also a new wisdom that has entered and opened us. This seeing extends not only to our fellow human, but to everything around us. We are born again! It is a whole new life, and it is very wonderful. As mentioned earlier, even if you do not reach this peak experience, this wonderful unfolding of the inner self, you can still find much peace by simply sitting quietly and breathing calmly. This is a renewing process for your whole being. Each time you sit, you are that much closer to your ultimate goal.

Seven Tips for a Successful Meditation

You are more likely to have a successful meditation if you try to following tips:

- Have a special room or a private corner. It will give you a feeling of special purpose and add atmosphere.

- Try adding symbolic articles to your meditation space, such as a statue, incense, a candle, or maybe a flower.

- The stillness of the day is a good time to practice. At sunrise or sunset, the whole universe is at peace. Our minds are fairly still when we arise, so generally sunrise is considered to be best time to meditate. Sunrise also brings a certain calm and strength for the day ahead.

- Be habitual about your meditation practice. Make it a habit, and have a regular time to sit. You will find that you are more ready for it. You'll begin to anticipate the *doing* of it. Your mind and body will react to being programmed. Therefore, your practice will soon become automatic.

- Our mind generally works better if we sit in meditation. We tend to associate kneeling with praying and lying down with falling asleep. Sit to your awakening. If you have trouble sitting on the floor, sit in a chair. Simply remember to keep your back straight, not stiff, and to close your eyes.

- Try meditating outdoors. It is like getting away from the world. If you are in tune with nature, you'll feel a oneness with the infinite. Did you ever stand outside on a starry night, look up, and completely forget about yourself? Did you feel as though you were a part of all the heavens and the stars? *That's* what mediation is like. A good way to meditate outside is to sit with your back to a tree and tune in to the tree for a moment. If you are really open to the experience, you will feel the aliveness of the tree. Our blood circulates through our body like sap moves through a tree. You will feel the life of it. Something about a tree opens to us when we open to it. It is very relaxing. Try it.

- Remember that meditation is not copping out of life, but moving into the reality and the truth of life.

Continuities

Begin by closing your eyes, and breathing deeply. As you inhale, your stomach pushes outward. As you exhale, your stomach falls inward. Tell yourself that this is your time to let go, to relax, to just be. You are free of stress and free of thoughts. You are in this moment. Now it's time to practice continuities in the order listed.

Seated Continuity

1. Fingers (Raindrops) #100
2. Head Turn and Bend to Side #118
3. Neck Roll #7
4. Turtle #93
5. Shoulder Lift and Roll #8
6. Stretch/Open Eyes/Yawn #130
7. Sitting Backward Stretch #36
8. Butterfly and Advanced #19
9. Reverse Balance Leg Lift #104

Reclining/Seated Continuity

1. Half and Full Bow #44
2. Half and Full Locust #45
3. Infant Posture and Stretch #17

Standing Continuity

1. Skeleton #18
2. Airplane #37
3. Standing Twist #38
4. Sun Worship/Sun Salutation #64
5. Centered Triangle #74
6. Holding the Balloon #116

 New Postures

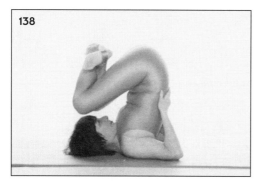

137. Butterfly Variation.

Sit in Butterfly position (#19) with your knees bent and the soles of your feet together. Inhale, place your hands behind your head, and interlace your fingers. Exhale, gently twist to the left, and place your right elbow on your left knee. Inhale to raise your body. Exhale, twist to the right, and place your left elbow on your right knee. Inhale and raise your body.

138. Plow (Cross Leg Variation).

This is an easier version of Plow posture (#40) for those who have difficulty with full extensions or difficulty breathing in full Plow posture. Lie on the floor with your legs raised, as if you are preparing to lower them in Plow position. Support your back with your hands. Cross your legs at the knees. On your exhalation, bend your knees and lower them to your chest. Inhale and straighten your legs up. You may also alternate lowering your knees to your left shoulder, then to your right shoulder.

139. Pelvic Leg Lift.

This posture may be used as an alternative to Pelvic Lift (#41), and as an inverted posture to be practiced after Plow positions (#40, #138, #152). Assume raised Pelvic Lift. Inhale and release your right heel. Raise your right leg up and straighten it out. Exhale, lower your leg, and grasp your heel with your hand again. Inhale and repeat this movement for your left leg.

Relaxation/Meditation: Beginning Meditation

The first step of meditation is to sit for a few minutes with your eyes closed. Your breathing should be relaxed, smooth, soft, and flowing. The second step is a little more difficult—emptying your mind! Meditation is not truly doing anything; rather, it is not doing. It is simply to be. "To be" means to be detached and attached at the same time. You become detached from personal involvement of anything that takes place around you, and detached from any thoughts that insist on passing through and flooding your mind. However, in meditation you will also remain attached, in the sense that you are wholly aware of, and in, this moment. If we could all become a lake or even a small pond for a moment, we would have a better understanding of how we should be. We must reflect, but not truly take on what touches us, like the water responds to the moon, the Wei Wu Wei—action without re-action. When we are detached we make no distinction between good or bad; everything just is. In time, even that much disappears. You will want to choose the meditation method that best suits you. Some are taught to sit with the firmness of a mountain. Others imagine a massive oak tree, deeply rooted, with a strong, straight trunk, mighty, majestic, and unmoving. Then, they become it. If you too might want to choose to meditate on an image; then, following your breath in and out. Feel your breath enter your nostrils, fill your being, and flow gently outward once more. Instead of following your breath, you might prefer to repeat a mantra to yourself, over and over again, something simple, such as OM, peace, peace, peace.

For a simpler meditation, exhale and feel the vibration of your humming. You might decide that you would rather listen very intently to the silence. If a sound comes through, don't try to name it. Simply continue to listen to the silence as though you might hear the most important message of your life, and you will. Choose whatever meditation you think might best suit you, and try it now. (Pause.)

Do you feel content just as you are at this moment? What is there to be desired that this moment does not hold? When you feel this inner peace, this quiet joy, could you possibly wish for more? This moment is special because you are not dependent on anything or anyone. Everything is wholly yours, an unending source of peace. You must only open yourself to it and allow it to happen. Try to truly feel it for just a moment more. (Pause.)

Now, you may lie down, stretch out, and relax. If you opened yourself to your sitting and aware of the experience, your body should already be relaxed as you lie down. It feels very light, almost nonexistent, and the inner you is smiling. We can only feel this way when we truly put the ego self aside, which we must do to enter meditation.

In your sitting, you come to a quiet knowing, a new understanding of life. A new dimension expands before you and in you. When you return to your usual routines, everything is different because you are different. Your inner attitude changes. While your outward movements remain the same, you perform them with a new sense of hearing and feeling and seeing and knowing. You throw your blinders away and raise your face to the sun! (Pause.)

Think about how you feel right now. Do you feel rested, peaceful, content? Are you still smiling inwardly? Are you in your moment? This moment is the pause that truly refreshes, renews, revives, restores, and reunites us to the essence of what and who we truly are. (Pause.)

Always remember that your body needs movement, your mind needs rest, and your spirit needs inspiration. When you combine these three principles, you become a whole person. To be whole is to be holy!

Welcome yourself back to aliveness with a gentle stretch and your private affirmation: "My body is rested and my mind is peaceful. I feel whole and complete just as I am at this moment, and this moment is complete." Fully stretch. Yawn your release, and smile to your wholeness.

If you are too blind to see God in the sunrise and sunset
and in all that lies between,
then pause long enough to FEEL the holy,
the rain upon your face,
the sun's warmth, the cool of the breeze.
The message can be received as simply as hugging a tree.
And, it is signed: GOD!
Shanti — Shanti — Shanti — Peace — Peace — Peace

ADVANCED LEVEL 3 LESSON 3

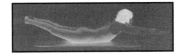

In order to be in the now, we must pay attention to the moment. However, few of us have such attention. When we dedicate our attention, it is usually of short duration, spasmodic, intermediate, and passive. One reason behind this lack of attention is that we think about our living, instead of living our thinking. The point of life becomes second hand or second rate. Whereas, if we enlighten each moment with attention, we do not need to search for enlightenment. All spiritual paths and teachings have different names for attention or mindfulness, but none have been able to define it totally. Why? Attention is so closely linked with being and equally indefinable. Regardless of the given name, the inner state of mindfulness remains the same.

The Path to the Now

Reality can only be found in the now, in the moment. You will not find it in the past or in the future because these don't exist. You must pay attention to now.

The following suggestions will help you on your journey:

- True attention lets us see all things transfigured.

- True attention allows for a life free of boredom.

- True attention is life lived and experienced to its fullest.

- Opening to the force of attention evokes a sense of wholeness and equilibrium.

- Attention is not only a form of meditation. It is a transmission. In other words, our vibrations become stronger and more powerful.

- True attention is being aware of the silence between, as well as the sound of the notes or of the spoken word. In listening to someone speak, be aware of the silence between the words, as well as the words.

True attention is the key to all the elements in the path of the now. It also facilitates formal sitting meditation by training our mind to pay complete attention. The pause in life is very important. When you hold or pause in a certain position, you experience one of the most important times in your life. Your body is talking to you and telling you where it is strong, where it is weak, and what it needs. You are learning about yourself. The pause of the stretch, that pause between breaths is extremely exciting. You inhale and, naturally, your breath pauses, and then, you exhale. The paradox is that during the pause between breaths, at the very moment when there is no life, per se, you feel more alive than when you are truly in the breath. Let this happen to you sometime.

 # Continuities

Sit fairly straight, but not stiff. Simply close your eyes and breathe deeply, allowing all stress to leave with every exhalation. Allow new awareness to enter you with every inhalation. Breathe. When you are ready, begin practicing the following continuities in the order listed.

Reclining Continuity

1. Infant Posture and Stretch #17
2. Upper Body Stress Release #88
3. Lion #11
4. Gate I #69
5. Gate II #70
6. Elimination #9
7. Camel #29
8. Raised Bow #65
9. Forearm-Wrist Stretch #61
10. Swan #22
11. Floating Swan #23
12. Balance on Fours #24
13. Cat Variations #28

Standing Continuity

1. Toes, Flat, Chair, Tree #15
2. Standing Waist Roll #51
3. Windmill #52
4. Sun Worship/Sun Salutation #64
5. Balanced Breath #67

New Postures

140. Weightless Arm Lift.

Assume a comfortable standing position with your arms at your sides. Inhale, rise up on your toes, and lift your arms to the ceiling. Hold this posture for as long as it is comfortable. Exhale, lower your heels to the floor and your arms to your sides.

141. Rama's Easy Pose.

Assume a comfortable standing position with your arms by your sides. Inhale, rise up on your toes, and lift your arms out to the sides. Exhale as you lower your heels to the floor. Bend your elbows and bring your hands to your chest, then lower your hands to your sides.

142. Bouncing on Knee Breath.

Stand comfortably with your arms at your sides. Inhale as you raise your left leg, take a step forward and bend your left knee. Very gently and loosely bounce up and down. Exhale as you lower your body, and inhale as you raise your body. Your right heel may slightly leave the floor as you bounce up and down. Repeat this movement for your opposite leg. The goal of this posture is to get your blood circulating throughout your body.

Relaxation/Meditation: Tree and Sand

Stand with your eyes closed. Breathe and relax. You are in a centered stance with your feet below your hips. Do not lock your knees. Your back is straight, but not stiff. Your head rests lightly on your neck.

Just as the oak tree draws energy and life from the earth and the sky, you too will try to feel this energy. Begin with your feet. Every time you inhale, feel the energy of the earth flowing upward through your feet. Try this first. (Pause.)

Can you increase this energy? On your next inhalation, let this energy rise even further, through your feet and up through your legs. Picture this energy as a very fine mist, if you wish. Try it now. (Pause.)

Keep following your inhalation and feel the energy enter your feet, travel up through your legs, and enter just below your waist. You can do it. Do it now. (Pause.)

These next inhalations will truly energize a vital part of your trunk—your navel and solar plexus. Try it now. (Pause.)

Feeling almost completely energized, you will bring this energy, this life force, to its final level. This time, when you inhale, you will feel the energy pass through your throat and enter the top of your head. You will feel totally energized and light. Do it now. (Pause.)

Experience, with each inhalation, how the earth energy enters the soles of your feet and, slowly and comfortably, rises and rises, up and up, right to the top of your head. Even though the energy is rising upward, and the upper part of your body feels light and alive, you still feel planted quite firmly from your waist down. Enjoy it for a few moments. (Pause.)

Whenever you want to revive yourself after a hard and stressful day, even though your mind may tell you to flop down and watch T.V, let your inner self remind you to stand as you are right now. Keep your body centered so that the energy can travel freely upward. Do not make your breathing too forceful or too demanding on the pull upward. When you feel energized and relaxed, simply stand there for a few moments and absorb this feeling, before releasing yourself from the position. (Pause.)

Now, you may release yourself from this position. Gently lower your body and center yourself on the floor. Release and relax your body. Close your eyes, and breathe slowly. (Pause.)

As you lie on the floor, picture yourself getting away from it all. You've gone to your own private beach. You walk down toward the water's edge. Feel the tiny grains of sand release under the weight of your body. Feel the grip of your toes and the grains of sand massaging your feet gently. Then, you stop. Work your toes in and out of the soft white sand. It invites you to sit down, and you do. Reaching out, you take a handful of sand, and let it drain between your fingertips back to its resting place. It is warm, soothing to the touch. You take another handful of sand and repeat the process a few more times. Your knees are bent. Your forehead rests on your knees. Your arms are relaxed by your sides, and your hands rest in the warm sand. It is so peaceful. You can feel the warm sun on your back and the gentle breeze from the water's edge. You can hear the waves washing ashore, splashing in and out, in and out, like a softly hummed mantra. Finally, you lie back on the warm sand and let the hum cradle you to a gentle, restful sleep. Stay in this place, and enjoy it. (Pause.)

The sound of the sandpiper calls you to awake once more. Smile to yourself for having rested peacefully, and begin your first stretch to the words of your affirmation: "My body is relaxed and my mind is peaceful. I feel whole and complete just as I am at this moment, and this moment is perfect." It is time for your full stretch, your welcomed yawn, and your contented smile. You are home.

Awareness is your only real connection with the present.
If you don't have this now, what DO you have?
Shanti—Shanti—Shanti—Peace—Peace—Peace

ADVANCED LEVEL 3 LESSON 4

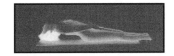

It is difficult to look at ourselves in fearless honesty, uninfluenced by ideas and images of what we are, should be, or have been told we should be. Outwardly, we might feel as though we are defying some sort of social authority. Inwardly, we question our own being. Yet, only with this insight can our mind begin to free itself from its conditioning and can the true spirit of us come to life.

The Experience of Life

Our reaction to life is generally programmed. We respond out of memory in both action and language. In other words, we react automatically to life and to the moment, rather than spontaneously. Why do we do this? The familiar feels more comfortable, easier, and safer. You can continue to believe the varied definitions of "truth" you might hear. However, you could instead experience truth firsthand.

The following story illustrates this experience. A very rich emperor loved blueberries and looked for a man who would know the most about them. He spoke with one man who had read many books about blueberries: how to cultivate them and in what conditions, the right season, and so forth. He was considered an authority. The second man had never studied blueberries and was untrained. When asked by the emperor about blueberries, the first man went into great detail about how to determine the very best blueberry; the second man simply plucked the berries from the vine and experienced it. Who do you think knew more about the blueberry?

Experiencing life is attention to life. Attention to life is being spontaneous. When we cease to react to the images in our memory, our senses act as a whole, and we see the whole picture. Ask yourself the following: Am I willing to question all my past opinions, information, and points of view? Am I willing to break the link of thoughts, impressions, feelings, and emotions that my parents and others have inflicted on me, which have all become my ways? Will I stay clothed in comfort and in the familiar, or will I strip myself of the old and dress in the new? I am not suggesting that everything others have taught you is wrong, and that you should wipe out this information. I am simply recommending that you see this world through *your* eyes, and experience it with *your* senses.

Learn to be with the moment, whether it is the wind blowing, the rain on your face, a baby crying, your stomach growling, or a deep sigh. All are new each moment, and you cannot be bored. The new is not boring, only our memory leads us to believe that something is boring. Our awareness to life makes everything new, exciting, and meditative.

Doesn't it sound exciting? Are you ready to bring this into your life? Are you ready to live this way? Do you want to take the giant leap? The choice is yours.

 # Continuities

Begin with your breathing. Relax into this moment, free of stress and thought, only aware of the now and of each breath you are about to take. Close your eyes. When you are centered and relaxed, practice the following continuities in the order listed.

Standing Continuity

1. Standing Backward Stretch #50
2. Tension Mill #92
3. Back and Hips Rotations #96
4. Standing Hip Strengthener #71
5. Sun Worship/Sun Salutation #64

Reclining Continuity

1. Fish #5
2. Tension Twist #124
3. Plow and Variations #40
4. Pelvic Lift #41
5. Three-Quarter Shoulder Stand #42
6. Upper and Lower Rolls #43
7. Head to Knee and Pull #6

Seated Continuity

1. Sitting Leg Stretch #27
2. Anterior Stretch #39
3. Lotus Relaxed Posture #57

Standing Continuity

1. Weightless Arm Lift #140
2. Rama's Easy Pose #141
3. Bouncing on Knee Breath #142

New Postures

143. Carefree.

Assume a comfortable standing position. Inhale and raise your arms out to yours sides at shoulder height. Keep your shoulders high and make quick chopping motions backward. Exhale on each backward movement, and inhale on each forward movement. Your breathing will be as rapid as the movement of your arms. Exhale and slowly lower your arms. The purpose of this posture is to get your circulation moving.

144. Strengthening Nerve Breath.

Assume a comfortable standing position. Inhale, bend your elbows, and raise the lower part of your arms up and in front to about waist high. Your palms should face upward. Make your hands into fists. Move both arms backward and forward, very quickly and very vigorously. Exhale on each backward movement, and inhale on each forward movement. Your breathing will be as rapid as the movement of your arms. Exhale, and slowly lower your arms. The purpose of this posture is to get your circulation moving.

145. Forward Swing Breath.

Stand comfortably. Inhale and lift your arms over your head. Exhale and very slowly bend forward, down to the floor, and hang there. When you are ready, inhale, and slowly lift your body. Allow your inhalation to lift your body. Exhale and relax. The purpose of this posture is to get circulation to your head.

Relaxation/Meditation: The Chakras

In yoga, we refer to the various centers of our being as chakras. Our chakras are located throughout our body. Kundalini Yoga concentrates on opening the chakras by using several breathing techniques. It takes much time, practice, and dedication to learn how to open all our chakras. This relaxation will give you a basic overview. Each chakra has its own color and a certain number of lotus petals. Each petal contains letters of the Sanskrit alphabet, which form the sound of a mantra. Sound and breath work together in the charkas, and each chakra has its own position in the body. By associating yourself with individual chakra colors and positions, you can begin to familiarize yourself with their existence and your relationship to each.

Make yourself comfortable on the floor in a sitting or kneeling position. Feel centered, released, and relaxed. Close your eyes. Your breathing is smooth and effortless. In this visualization, try to feel the color and location of your chakra, what it represents—its quality.

Begin with the first chakra. Its color is pink and has a red energy to it. It is located at the base of your spine. It represents vitality and earthly love. How does it feel to you? (Pause.)

The second chakra is also of earthly vitality and courage. The color is orange, and is located in the genital area. Orange. Can you feel its energy? (Pause.)

Move upward to your third chakra. It is golden yellow and located at your navel. It is associated with the solar plexus and earthly wisdom. How does this feel to you? (Pause.)

Your fourth chakra is your heart chakra, and its color is green. This chakra is for concentration. It represents maternal love and earthly healing. Can you feel its vibration and its quality? (Pause.)

Your fifth chakra is in your throat area, and its color is light blue. This color is one of mental healing and articulation. Can you become one with it? (Pause.)

Your sixth level chakra is often referred to as your third eye. It is located in the center of your forehead. Its color is indigo blue. It represents mental healing, and the opening of the psychic center. Much calm is needed to open this chakra. It might be easier for you to feel this chakra if you are already familiar with the third eye. (Pause.)

Your seventh chakra—the crown chakra—is located on the top of your head. Its color is violet for spiritual health and enlightenment. It is a very pretty chakra with its thousand lotus petals, symbolizing the infinite. Would it not be nice to truly experience this one? Just try it. (Pause.)

Stay a little longer in this chakra center, and truly try to feel it. (Pause.)

Keep your eyes closed, and gently lower your body to the floor—centered, loose and limp, released and relaxed. Each center, each chakra, is much like a telephone center with many different wires coming in and going out of it. Just as we cannot see the electricity in those wires, we cannot see the prana energy created by our breathing, but we can feel it.

What area and color were the most comfortable for you? Are you still a rainbow of colors? It might take time for you to settle into just one color or no color, only the pure white light of your being. We are beings of light, pure, precious, and perfect at this moment. We come to this realization through deep meditation. We no longer simply look in from the outside, but, rather, we look out from the inside. (Pause.)

Come out with your first gentle stretch and your affirmation: "My body is relaxed and my mind is peaceful. I am whole and complete just as I am at this moment, and this moment is perfect." Fully stretch and awaken. Yawn and smile joyously. You are home.

A fool wastes his precious life reliving the past or fantasizing about the future.
Life and living are now and only now.
Eternity is made up of "nows."
By missing one, we miss eternity.
Shanti—Shanti—Shanti—Peace—Peace—Peace

ADVANCED LEVEL 3 LESSON 5

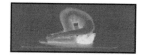

editation is sometimes difficult because it requires that we set the ego aside. We are so attached to our ego, so dependent upon it, that we become afraid to let it go. Actually, it is the ego is holding us prisoner. You shouldn't let the ego keep you from entering into meditation. When you come out of your meditation, your ego will be waiting for you. However, after you have touched the inner you, you will have no need to care for your ego. Why? Because in meditation you will have touched the paradise of the perfect, precious, inner you. Compared to that, the ego has very little to offer. And no one wants to miss paradise!

Spontaneous and Deliberate Concentration

Crystallized meditation is a very deep, refined meditation that is only possible after the groundwork of concentration is established. There are two specific kinds of concentration. One is spontaneous and automatic, while the other is deliberate and controlled. Spontaneous concentration occurs when our mind focuses voluntarily, because it wants to, and offers no resistance. Our mind follows or obeys a strong, emotional motivation. For instance, we might become engrossed or spellbound by a piece of music or a majestic oak tree.

Deliberate concentration is has very little emotional urge or desire behind it. Because this can be unattractive to our mind, our mind will try to escape by interjecting distracting thoughts. To overcome our mind's tenacity, we must pull our mind back, again and again, if we wish to obtain a higher plane of consciousness. Unfortunately, our nature doesn't always have the enthusiasm to pursue higher aspirations. Sometimes our nature is much like a child who would rather play, than work at some form of mental advancement. Just as the child evades the work, our mind places distractions in our path. The actions of both the child and mind call for discipline.

Many techniques can be used in training your concentration. You can try to look at something for a few minutes, and then write down every detail that you can remember. Another practice is to create a mental picture, and then immediately dissolve it. A third technique is visualization. All three methods take practice, desire, dedication, and discipline.

Assume that you've been working on your concentration, and you feel that you've been doing fairly well. Suppose for a minute that you are sitting in meditation and asked to hold a small bowl of water in your hands. The bowl has a pinhole in the bottom where the water slowly drips out. You continue to sit, while the water drips, until finally the bowl is empty. What do you do? Do you place the bowl on the floor when the water is gone? If you choose to set the bowl down, you have set a time limit on your meditation and were not truly concentrating and meditating. You allowed your mind to distract you. If instead of setting the bowl down, you asked yourself: "What bowl?" Then you were concentrating and meditating.

In meditation, there is no time. The concept of no time keeps many people from practicing meditation because they fear that they will not be able to come out of the meditation. However, this is not true. Our innate being will always take care of us. If decide to sit in meditation for fifteen, twenty, thirty minutes, or however long you choose, you inner being will bring you back. However, if you stay in contact with that message center, then you will not enter meditation and will create an attachment for mind.

Continuities

Begin by breathing. Empty your mind of all outside influences, all stress, all frustrations and fears, all those things that the ego keeps handing you. Put it all aside, and touch the inner you. Touch this moment, this experiencing, this very breath. As you inhale, your stomach pushes outward. Exhale, and your stomach settles back in. Relax, and close your eyes. When you are ready to begin, practice the following continuities in order listed.

Reclining Continuity

1. Dreaming Dog #1
2. Lie and Stretch #2
3. Leg Raise I and II #3
4. Reverse Bow I and II #4
5. Ceiling Walk and Cross #34
6. Lying Knee to Head #31
7. Forward Boat #33

Seated Continuity

1. Full Rolls and Balance #26
2. Rowing #53
3. Sitting Twist Swing #54
4. Sitting Mill #55
5. Side Scissors #68
6. Side Scissors Variation #102

Standing Continuity

1. Standing Wall-Ceiling #30
2. Triangle Variations #125
3. Sun Worship/Sun Salutation #64
4. Pivot and Push #106
5. Jonathan Balance #73

New Postures

146. Rabbit.

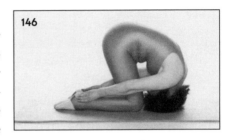

Start in basic Infant pose (#17) with your arms at your sides and your head to the floor in front of your knees. Take hold of your heels. Inhale and slowly roll your buttocks up in the air. All your weight is on your knees. As your buttocks are raised, your head position will automatically change so that more of your head is resting on the floor. There should be no weight on your neck or head. Your back and neck are curved. The purpose of this posture is to increase the circulation to your neck and face area and to release tension. Hold the posture for as long as you are comfortable. Exhale to lower your body.

147. Yoga Supported Back Bend.

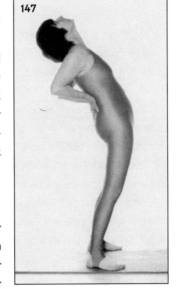

This is for individuals who have difficulty with unsupported backward bending postures. Stand with your feet comfortably apart and your arms by your sides. Inhale and place the palms of your hands on your back at about waist level. Exhale and gently lean back as far as it is comfortable. Use your hands to support your back. Inhale to return to an upright position.

148. QiGong Leg/Arm Warm-up.

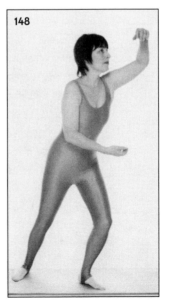

Stand with your feet apart and under your hips. Your arms are relaxed at your sides. Turn out your toes slightly. Slowly shift all of your weight to your left leg and slightly bend your left knee. At the same time, while bending your body slightly forward, slowly bring your right arm across the front of your body so that your hand is slightly above your left knee with your palm facing upward. In addition, at the same time, your left arm rises up and over your head, with your palm facing down to the top of your head. This is all one slow movement. Slowly bring your body back to center and repeat the posture for your opposite side. This pose should be practiced three times each way.

 ## Relaxation/Meditation: The Now

In this meditation, you will visit the now. Instead of trying to escape the ego self, as you usually try to do in meditation, you will now truly get in touch with yourself. Perhaps, for the first time, you will understand yourself more thoroughly. What is it that keeps after us and disturbs our peace?

Make yourself comfortable for this exploring adventure. Center your body to the floor. Relax all your muscles. Don't hold anything back or up. Let go and sink down with each exhalation. (Pause.)

Begin with the premise that our life is better witnessed with an awareness of opposites, like our in-breath and out-breath. For example, you feel the pleasure of relaxing only after you move your body through your postures. We are not always able to thoroughly experience the opposites of life because of society's emphasis on constant activity. We are always being pushed to go and to do. We are rarely encouraged to stop, to be still, to pause, to be!

How much of this day did you spend in the now? Answer yourself honestly. Get to really know yourself, the why of you. Did you sit and do nothing? (Pause.)

If not, why? (Pause.)

When an emotion hit you, did you stop and try to understand it and its origin? (Pause.)

Did you take the time to enjoy the sensations of your connection to life? (Pause.)

Did you truly smell the morning breeze? (Pause.)

Did you truly feel your morning stretch? (Pause.)

Did you truly taste your morning morsel of food? (Pause.)

How did the sunrise look this morning? (Pause.)

Did you see the stars last night? (Pause.)

In order to understand your connection to your life, you must be honest with yourself. (Pause.)

Did you balance your doing with your not doing, today? Did pause as well as push? (Pause.)

In order to reach harmony, balance, and the joy of living, you must give into the hum of your being, like a cat gives into a purr. Do you feel like humming now? (Pause.)

If some of this practice doesn't come easily to you, and, in the beginning, it probably won't, then take spot checks on yourself at different times of the day. Stop and ask yourself: "How's my breathing?" Check to see if it is relaxed, full, and deep. If it isn't, then stop and fix it! Stop and take a few deep breaths. You can ask yourself: "Am I moving, standing, and sitting balanced?" If the answer is no, fix it! Don't be afraid to give yourself some positive thoughts and repeat affirmations throughout the day. Repeat these to yourself now:

- I am feeling calm and relaxed.
- I am going with the flow.
- I am in my moment.

- I feel light and free.
- I feel whole and complete.
- There is nothing that I desire at this moment.
- I feel connected with everything about me.
- I feel connected with my higher self.
- It is good to be alive.
- Life is a celebration!

How do you feel? If you kept yourself open to these positive suggestions, you should be feeling pretty good about yourself and about life. By reaffirming these thoughts, life will improve for you. You will have a new love for yourself, along with a new understanding and a new acceptance of yourself. Take the leap, not just of faith in yourself, but, more importantly, of belief in yourself. You are only limited by thought. When you truly believe you can do something, then it is done!

Believe that you can gently stretch yourself back to aliveness. Affirm: "My body is relaxed and my mind is peaceful. I am whole and complete just as I am at this moment, and this moment is perfect." Stretch fully and release a yawn and a grateful smile. You're home.

The first time you truly SEE,
the ordinary becomes
EXTRA-ORDINARY!
Shanti—Shanti—Shanti—Peace—Peace—Peace

ADVANCED LEVEL 3 LESSON 6

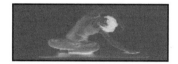

As an advanced yoga student, you understand that the success of your concentration and meditation does not depend on how your body sits but on how your mind is set. Regular daily meditation, even for as little as five or ten minutes a day, is crucial for a successful practice. Our difficulty in controlling our mind can be compared to folding a piece of leather. Folding it one way is fairly easy, but the difficulty arises when we try to fold it in the opposite direction. For countless ages, our minds have been turned outward. Now, we are trying to turn our minds inward. It is not an easy task. To some it might seem impossible, but with patience it can happen.

The Union of Meditation

There is a meditation room in the United Nations building in New York called a room of silence. Light streams into this room as from the unseen Source overhead. The greatest of men and women have known the value of meditation in their lives, from Buddha, to Jesus, to Gandhi. They knew the power, the worth, the satisfaction, and the peace of meditation. Meditation creates a union and a sense of oneness at the center of our existence. At times, our mistake is in seeking separateness by flaunting our individuality and wanting to be different, special, or unique from everyone else. We say: "See how wonderful *I* am!"

The biggest mistake that we make is alienating ourselves from nature. We all have experienced moments when we have felt a part of the whole. In these fleeting moments, such as standing outside on a starry night, our higher consciousness is trying to seep through. Unfortunately, we tend to ignore it. The next time you find yourself outside, take a moment and sit. Look around you, and see and feel the single petal on a flower. Focus your full attention on a bird singing. Feel its joy and be as it is. Bring your awareness to a single blade of grass, to the drop of dew on its tip, and see the ocean reflected there. How are you different from the flower, the bird, and the grass? Are you not also rooted in the earth? Are you not also reaching heavenward? Eternity is made up of now and now and now. Isn't your life a series of nows? Why should you separate yourself from the wholeness, the oneness—from eternity?

Continuities

Sit and simply breath for a moment. Empty yourself of all outer things, and tune in on your inner being. Close your eyes. When you are ready to being, practice the following continuities in order listed.

Seated/Reclining Continuity

1. Fingers (Raindrops) #100
2. Head Turn and Bend to Side #118
3. Neck Roll #7
4. Turtle #93
5. Shoulder Lift and Roll #8
6. Yoga Triceps Stretch #113
7. Stretch/Open Eyes/Yawn #130
8. Reverse Balance Leg Lift #104
9. Round Rolls #131
10. Half and Full Bow #44
11. Half and Full Locust #45
12. Infant Posture and Stretch #17

Standing Continuity

1. Standing Head to Knee #13
2. Wood Chop #14
3. Bear Walk and Lower #47
4. Sun Worship/Sun Salutation #64
5. Lunge Coordination Walk #114
6. Tree Balance #95

New Postures

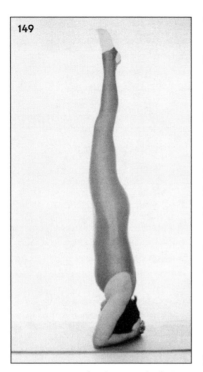

149. Headstand.

Until you are experienced with this posture, it is important that you always have a teacher, or someone trained in yoga practice, standing next to you. Assume Hare posture (#32). Your hands should be about six inches from a wall. Remember, it is important that not to move your elbows as you get into position. If you move your arms inward, you will not have a solid base and may fall to the side. If you move your arms outward, you will place weight on your head or your neck, which is also incorrect. Raise your hips so that you are standing on your toes. Walk forward to bring your toes as close to your body as you can. Bending your knees, bounce gently on your toes until you can bend your knees and bring both feet off the floor at the same time. Your knees remain bent. Slowly straighten your knees and raise your legs upward. The wall is behind you, so you will not fall backward. If you wish, you may rest your feet on the wall to get a better feeling of security. To come down, bend your knees and draw them down to your chest. Straighten your knees and lower your feet until your toes touch the floor. It is important to lower yourself down slowly, to keep from landing with your knees to the floor. Do not stand up immediately or you will feel dizzy. Once you have lowered your toes to the floor, rest in this position for a few moments. Then, inhale and raise your body to an upright kneeling position. You may not want to try this posture if you have neck problems.

150. Ascending Breath.

Take a balanced stance with your feet below your hips. Your arms are at your sides. Inhale, bend your elbows, and raise your hands to waist level with your palms facing downward. Exhale, bend your knees, and push down with your hands. Inhale, straighten your knees, and push your hands out to your sides. Exhale, bend your knees, and push your hands down. Inhale, straighten your knees, and push your hands up over your head. Exhale and let your hands float down to your sides. This is a very relaxing posture. Try to do the complete rotation three times.

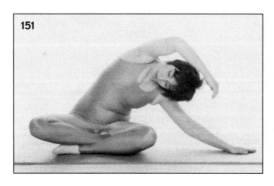

151. Sitting Side Stretch.

Sit cross-legged on the floor. Lean to the left and place your left palm flat on the floor. Bend to the left, starting from your waist. Inhale, lift your chest high, and stretch your right arm over your head. Keep your buttocks on the floor. Your body is supported by your left arm. Breathe deeply. On your exhalation lower your body and right arm, and return to a centered sitting position. Repeat for the other side of your body.

Relaxation/Meditation: The Fountain of Light

Your success in relaxation and meditation basically depends on your openness and participation in each journey you take. Let me tell you the story of the fountain of light: Several individuals go to the fountain of light in their meditations. Each one approaches it differently, even though all have an equal thirst for it. Some only dip into it lightly, and quickly depart from it. Others stay longer and fill themselves a little more before leaving. But then, someone approaches the fountain with the lightness, the trust, and the innocent faith of a child, and, lo and behold, this person jumps right into the center of the fountain. When he departs, there is a new sparkle in his eyes and new laughter on his lips. My question to you is: Will you jump in? Will you fill and reward yourself?

Begin by relaxing your body to the floor—centered, released, and relaxed. Empty your mind of everything but this experiencing, this precious moment of now. Let your breath take you down, down, and deeper within yourself—your real self. Do this now. (Pause.)

Learning to let go of the things that prevent you from finding the joy and the bliss you desire can be as simple as making a choice, a positive decision to change. You must allow yourself to take that leap of faith and jump in! Think for a moment: What is it that is stopping you? Think about this now. (Pause.)

Imagine that you are writing your problem down on a piece of paper. (Pause.)

Don't try to push this thought or the problem aside. You'll get rid of it right now. (Pause.)

Picture your piece of paper poised a couple of feet above your closed eyes. Every time you exhale, picture a thin film of mist leaving you and traveling up to that piece of paper. The mist begins to surround the piece of paper like the film of a translucent bubble. Do this now. (Pause.)

Completely surround the piece of paper, and let the paper float freely within the bubble you have created. (Pause.)

It should be complete. On your next exhalation, set the bubble free and let it begin to drift upward. With each exhalation, let it continue to rise higher and higher. (Pause.)

This shouldn't be difficult. Breathe normally. The bubble is very light and will rise quite easily. Simply watch it do so. (Pause.)

The bubble is taking your problem with it. See it grow further and further away. (Pause.)

It is nearly out of sight, growing smaller and more distant, up and finally out of sight. Doesn't it feel good? Do you feel released? Do you feel free? You let this problem go for your self.

Every change, every choice we make is a step forward, even though it doesn't always seem so at the time. We are all exactly where we are supposed to be. The choices and changes that we make are the ones we should make at that particular time. If you are still in doubt, still holding back and holding on, then, simply watch the spot where that bubble disappeared. The magical, wonderful, and loving force that always watches over you will send a message back. Watch. (Pause.)

Keep watching and it will appear. Stay relaxed, trusting, and open. (Pause.)

Can you see it? It is the beautiful, translucent bubble drifting slowly down toward you, again. (Pause.)

See how it pauses above you once more? Do you see the paper inside? It's a message for you. Are you ready for it? If you are, see yourself reach up, burst the bubble, and take the piece of paper in your hands. Read it. (Pause.)

It says: "The fountain of light welcomes you. Your leap of faith will reward you with more love, more clarity, than you have ever witnessed before! Bathe within that light. Swim in it, as if propelled by a fuel of fins. Float in the froth of the surface. But always be in it and of it, whatever the level of your experience. You have claimed your inheritance." Is this what you read? This *is* the message. If you did not see it this time, it will be there next time, and the next time. Relax for a moment, and experience how you feel right now. (Pause.)

Come back to the room around you, to *this* experiencing. As you bring your body back to aliveness, stretch gently and affirm: "My body is relaxed and my mind is peaceful. I am whole and complete just as I am at this moment, and this moment is perfect!" Stretch into the full awareness of your body, your releasing yawn, and the new smile upon your lips. Welcome home!

Where can you find the sacred?
In birds and bears, dolphins and ducks,
rocks and rivers, fields and forest, streams and stars,
hills and havens, trees and trails.
When will you understand that?
You will understand when you have truly learned to SEE!
Shanti—Shanti—Shanti—Peace—Peace—Peace

ADVANCED LEVEL 3 LESSON 7

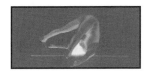

Nature is a very special friend. It can teach us many wonderful and useful things that help us grow, be more content, more connected with our natural essence, more spontaneous to life, and more complete. Unfortunately, we sometime don't listen to our friend. Can we learn to hear before it is too late?

Responsiveness

We have forgotten to be aware of the life beyond that which we are. Nature/humankind is but one movement, each an echo of the other. Nature/humankind is but one expression, even though consciousness draws it to itself in different realities. The ultimate intelligence—God, if you wish—is expressed in many forms and is not the sole privilege of humankind. In other words, intelligence is One in many physical identities. We live in a very hazy, distorted reflection of what truly is. When we look into the depths of water, we can see what is reflected all around. However, we don't realize that when we view all life around us directly, void of the water, that too is a reflection of the real world. Why? Because we are looking with expression, not with openness. Openness requires a certain amount of humility. Unfortunately, we often don't want to humble ourselves. Some of us have no trouble identifying with the animal kingdom. We talk to our animals. But very, few of us identify with the plant kingdom. Some of us have learned to talk to our house plants, but when was the last time we talked to a tree?

The way in which we perceive the things outside ourselves is a reflection of our inner nature. In life, we should always seek knowing, rather than knowledge. Knowledge is only a multitude of accumulated facts and second hand information that doesn't make us more evolved than the storehouse knowledge of a computer. Knowing, on the other hand, firsthand experience is the living world. Knowing is timeless and spaceless. It is bound by no laws. Knowing is information in movement, kept free and spontaneous. Life is not revealed by building up layer upon layer of stored information. Life is grasping each new now.

Life is learning to be responsive rather than reactive. Reactiveness is generally predictable, worn, dead, and automatic. Responsiveness is truer to the moment, to the situation, and is the result of this now. When you perceive the now—the is—you will find a moment of infinite tenderness and joy where you will not only hear the sound, but also the silence that surrounds it. You will not only see the form, but also the space of which it is formed. What an exciting experience this will be! It is worth every effort. It is a whole new aspect of life that more of us need to get in touch with.

 # Continuities

You are here, in the moment, grasping for it, and it is within your reach, now. You simply have to be open to it and allow it. Sit with expectation. Sit with innerness. Sit with peace. Sit and breathe, now. Close your eyes. When you are ready to begin, practice the following continuities in the order listed.

Reclining/Seated Continuity

1. Infant Posture and Stretch #17
2. Upper Body Stress Release #88
3. Lion #11
4. Gate I #69
5. Gate II #70
6. Elimination #9
7. Wheel #112
8. Raised Bow #65
9. Forward Frog #20
10. Swan #22
11. Floating Swan #23
12. Balance on Fours #24
13. Cat Variations #28

Standing Continuity

1. Airplane #37
2. Standing Twist #389
3. Kiss the Foot #25
4. Sun Worship/Sun Salutation #64
5. Headstand #14

New Postures

152. Plow Spread.

This is sometimes called Open Plow. Begin with Basic Plow posture (#40). Inhale and raise both legs upward. Exhale, as you lower your legs behind your head and open them as wide as you can. Place your toes on the floor. Your arms may support your back or remain at the sides of your body. Inhale, raise your legs, and bring them together. Exhale, as you slowly lower your buttocks and then your legs to the floor.

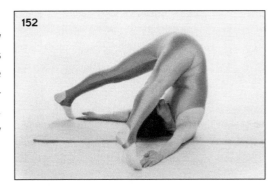

153. Lying Elbow to Crossed Knee.

Lie on the floor with your knees raised. Lift your right leg and cross your ankle over your left knee. Place your hands under your head with your fingers interlaced. Inhale, lift your body, and bring your left elbow to your right knee. Try not to bring your knee forward to meet your elbow. Exhale and lower yourself down. Repeat for the opposite side of your body.

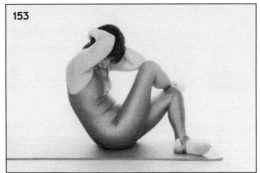

154. Tree Relaxation.

Take a comfortable stance with your feet slightly apart, and close your eyes. Imagine that your feet and legs are roots. Plant them firmly and feel them truly grounded. Feel your spine as the trunk of the tree, strong but flexible. Raise your arms and stretch them out as limbs, pointing slightly upward. Hold this position for a moment. You are no longer body. You are tree. Learn to react as one. Imagine a very strong wind passing through you. To come out of the posture, imagine that the wind is lessening; then, the wind ends. You are once again body. Relax your arms down to your sides.

Relaxation/Meditation: Yin/Yang Energy

When we use the word "opposites," we think of *contention*—a wedge of difference and separation. We do not think of *togetherness* and *harmony*. Yet, the whole universe, in order to exist, is based on this oppositeness. We must have night and day, hot and cold, wet and dry, and so forth. Although different, these complement one another and dependent upon one another. It is the balance of yin/yang. Nowhere is this dynamic better observed and experienced than in our breathing. Our in and out breath is yin/yang itself. Our right nostril is warmth and our left nostril is cold. When both are in balance—alternating breathing from one to the other—it becomes very calming, soothing, and restful.

This relaxation/meditation will explore this principle applied to the flow of your breath and the circulation of this energy flow throughout your body.

Begin on the upper part of your body. Sit comfortably with your back straight, but not stiff. Gently rest your head on your shoulders, and close your eyes. Take a few relaxing breaths. (Pause.)

Now that your breathing is relaxed and smooth, follow this flow of energy and really feel it taking place. With your next inhalation, feel the energy enter your left hand, travel up your left arm, cross over your shoulder and neck area.

As you exhale, feel this energy travel through your right shoulder, down the length of your right arm, through your right hand to your fingertips.

Then, start over again: in through the left and out through the right. Repeat this cycle for at least three rounds. After three rounds, feel the energy enter through the right, on your inhalation, and exit through the left, on your exhalation.

Practice this very slowly and with total awareness of what you are doing. Feel the gentle flow that is both energizing you and relaxing you. (Pause.)

When you have completed your cycles, you should feel greater harmony and more balance. Hold on to this feeling, and slowly lie back on the floor. Exhale, as you lower yourself down. Exhale your body into being released and relaxed; then, exhale further and further, allowing your body to go loose and limp, but still centered to its position.

You will now send yin/yang energy to every part of your being. When you are ready, inhale, and, this time, try to feel the energy enter your left foot and travel up your left leg to the base of your spine. As you exhale, feel this energy travel down your right leg to your right foot. Repeat this cycle three times.

On your next inhalation, reverse the energy flow. Feel the energy enter your right foot and travel upward. On your exhalation, feel it flow down your left leg to your left foot. Try this, now. (Pause.)

Move on the next step, which is the most enjoyable. You are going to bathe your entire upper body in this wonderful, soothing energy. Very simply, as you inhale, keep your awareness on the base of your spine. Feel the energy travel up your spine—the home of the yin/yang force—and flow right to the top of your head.

Exhale and feel this wonderful, calming flow pass gently over your face, your neck, your chest area, down to your abdomen, and out. Do not force this flow, simply witness it as it passes over you. Let it be as soft as the summer rain, warm and comfortable, soothing and relaxing, refreshing and reviving. Experience this, now. (Pause.)

Rest just as you are at this moment. Let nothing disturb you or interfere with this moment. Completely absorb this moment, become one with it—become it! It is home. It is the essence of you. It is the real you that always awaits your return, there anytime you open yourself to it. Become empty and allow it to be. Rest. (Pause.)

Imagine breathing twenty to twenty-three thousand times a day, then multiply this by the billions of inhabitants of this earth. Can you see the magnitude of energy that circulates through the universe, through all the universes? These interchanging energies circulate all around us, and we are a part of this moment. It has been said that nothing is ever lost, it merely changes. It is very likely that at some point in our lives, we have inhaled the energies of all who came before us—famous and infamous, holy and hellion, powerful and weak, blessed and bestial. What breath shall we send to those who follow us?

What will their inheritance be? We must make it pure and send it out with love from the very heart of your being!

It time to bring this new-found energy back to aliveness. Gently stretch yourself awake and affirm as always: "My body is relaxed and my mind is peaceful. I am whole and complete just as I am at this moment, and this moment is perfect!" With this new energy, allow yourself a good, long, gentle stretch and a fuller yawn, brighter, and happier smile. You are home!

When you are out in nature be on your best behavior,
as if you were a guest.
Because you ARE!
Different views of nature are different sightings of GOD!
Shanti—Shanti—Shanti—Peace—Peace—Peace

ADVANCED LEVEL 3 LESSON 8

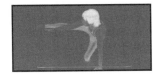

In order to develop a successful yoga practice, you can choose one of two paths: the formal way or the informal, natural, way. You might prefer the sitting way to the unseen, or the lived, way. Whichever you choose depends on the kind of person you are. You must discover what is better for you and what makes you feel more comfortable.

Choosing Your Path

Some of us are sitters, while others are livers (and I don't mean the kind you eat)! There are those who need or want the formality of sitting, and there are others who want to just be. Some people practice in both ways, which is even better. By the grace of God and by the grace of our own desire, all things are possible. Both paths are rewarding and bring growth. Both ways are easier to follow when you keep your body in shape and learn to control your breath. These practices are your chance to discover the real you and to base your life on a perfect balance of harmony. You will be able to wake from this dream of unreality and walk a life of total reality. These paths are your chance to witness and experience life with new understandings, to know heights of joy and peace and bliss, to see infinity in the finite and oneness in the ten thousand things. It is, indeed, heaven in the now. You can say "Yes!" to your practice and to your priceless inheritance.

Remember that life is a dance. In the beginning, we must follow the steps of others. However, there should come a time when we no longer need to follow others. Living is not a repetitive thing; it is ever-changing. We too must learn to change. Change to dance your own steps, even learn to lead, if you wish. But do not expect those you lead to follow you forever. Give them the freedom of their own steps, just as you have been given your freedom.

By following a non-rigid course, one that is spontaneous to life, we learn to be more surefooted, lighter on our feet. We can even learn to kick our heels high in the air. In the dance of life, some of us will waltz along, some of us foxtrot, some of us jig and twist, some pirouette or do-si-do. Some of us might miss a step and stumble, and that's okay. Each one of us will complete the dance of life at our own pace, with our own rhythm. We'll all deserve applause at the end. The only ones who will miss the applause are those who sit on the sidelines; those who refuse to join in the dance of life.

Follow and trust your own heart. In our everyday exchange with life, it is imperative that you use your mind. But when you want to follow your inner way, the higher way of consciousness, you must trust your heart. Your heart is very wise and has always protected you, loved you, cradled you, and held you. It will lead you on the right way this time, too. When you are out into the world, use your mind. When you go inward, follow your heart.

Continuities

Follow your breathing, and close your eyes. Let your body relax and your mind empty. Find the inner peace that is waiting for you right at this very moment. Then, practice the following continuities in the order listed.

Standing Continuity

1. Standing Backward Stretch #50
2. Tension Mill #92
3. Back and Hips Rotations #96
4. Standing Hip Strengthener #71
5. Wall-Ceiling Variation #85
6. Sun Worship/Sun Salutation #64
7. Pulsing #76

Reclining/Seated Continuity

1. Fish #59
2. Ceiling Walk and Cross #34
3. Plow and Variations #40
4. Pelvic Lift #41
5. Three-Quarter Shoulder Stand #42
6. Head to Knee and Pull #6
7. Anterior Stretch #3
8. Sitting Leg Stretch #27
9. Four-Limbed Stick Pose #75
10. Plank Pose #97
11. Infant Posture and Stretch #17

New Postures

155. Kneeling Side Kick.

Take the same kneeling position as Cat pose (#28), except that your fingers are facing forward. Shift all your weight to your left leg and left arm. Inhale and lift your right leg and right arm out to the side, at hip height. Exhale and lower your leg down. Repeat for the opposite side of your body.

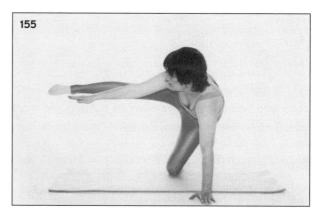

155

156. Circle Earth/Gather Clouds (energy).

This is the same posture as the Relaxed variation of Circle Earth/Gather Clouds (#109), but with a different purpose. Posture #109 is meant to relax your body, while this version is meant to energize your body and get your circulation moving. Instead of a gently swaying motion, in this version of the position, you will rock back and forth and make your arm movements more vigorous.

157. Golden Tai Chi.

Stand with your feet below your hips. Your hands are at about hip height at your sides. Inhale and slowly raise your arms to shoulder height in front of you with your fingers relaxed downward. Exhale by dropping your elbows, and draw your arms toward you so that your hands are at shoulder height. Resume regular breathing. Shift all your weight to your left leg. Step forward with your right foot, heel first, then drop your toes. As you begin the step, your right arm drops to a position slightly in front of your body and your right palm faces down. Your left arm circles up over your head with your palm facing down. Your arm movements should be completed at the same time as your right toe touches the floor. When the movement is complete, shift 70 percent of your weight to your right leg. Then, shift all your weight back to your left leg. Lift your right foot and return to the starting position, toe first, then drop your heel. As you begin the step, your arms return to the dropped elbow position with your hands in front of your shoulders. Your arm movements should be completed at the same time as your right heel touches the floor. Balance your weight, and lower your arms to your sides. Repeat this movement for the opposite side of your body. Once you have returned to the starting position, inhale and slowly raise your arms out to your sides and over the head with your fingers relaxed. Exhale and slowly lower your arms to your sides. As you bring your arms down, wiggle them as though they were raindrops. Inhale and raise your arms in front, again, with your fingers relaxed downward. Exhale and drop your elbows. Your hands are in front of your shoulders. Lower your arms to your sides, and relax your hands down.

Relaxation/Meditation: Reclaiming Your Inner Self

Anytime is a good time to connect with your inner self. Some of you might think that you are content and in touch with your inner self, that you're not missing out on what brings you joy.

If this sounds like you, think about the following questions. First you need to relax and center yourself. Lie down and release yourself to the floor. Center yourself comfortably, as you slowly lie down. Take a nice deep exhalation to release any the tightness and tension remaining in your body after your postures. Take another inhalation and a full exhalation to make sure that your body is loose and limp, released and relaxed. Softly close your eyes and give out a little sigh, if you wish. Your body likes to hear your sigh and will respond to it by letting go even further. Dwell on each question for a few seconds, then try to answer it as honestly as you can. Remember that the first answer that comes to mind is generally the right one. Your answer will tell you a lot about yourself and what you may be missing. Your honesty will bring you wholeness and happiness. If you are ready, we'll begin with the questions.

1. Have you lost your childhood spontaneity? If so, when? (Pause.)

2. When was the last time that you skipped through a pile of leaves and kicked them into the air? (Pause.)

3. When was the last time that you did something just to be silly? (Pause.)

4. When was the last time that you sang out loud to yourself, or whistled or hummed? (Pause.)

5. When was the last time that you truly saw, not only looked at, something in nature, and joined with it and felt it? (Pause.)

6. When was the last time that you were willing to simply sit quietly and listen to your inner voice, as you are doing now? (Pause.)

Our spontaneity to life sets us free, and brings us back to our naturalness. Instead of always *re*-acting to the things about us, we take action. Our action puts more life into our lives. The master within us comes into its own being.

When we skip or kick up our heels, we are saying that we're not weighted down by formality or the weight of our own being, both physical and mental.

Doing something that is silly, or what the world may call silly, might be important to our nature. It could help us release tension, give into the particular need of the moment, put a smile on our face, or bring laughter to our lips.

Singing out loud, whistling, or humming are expressions of joy. Have you ever sang, whistled, or hummed when you were depressed or angry? These are an expression of inner joy and, once we express them, they bring greater joy.

The healing and realizing of our true self is always found within our connection with nature. Nature is the greatest and wisest teacher.

Finally, sit quietly and become absorbed in the silence. This moment is when all questions end and all knowing begins. It is far more profound than the reading of any book, the listening of any voice, the learning that any teacher may impart. Everything that you need to know is already inside you. Your own master awaits your presence. Open yourself to it, as you have done in this relaxation.

The answers that you received in your private visitation with your being are known only to you, and you alone must decide the changes that you wish to make in your life.

It is time again to gently stretch yourself back to the room around you, to this experiencing, to this now. Begin your journey while you give yourself the affirmation: "My body is relaxed and my mind is peaceful. I am whole and complete just as I am at this moment, and this moment is complete." Stretch fully. Energize yourself with a yawn and a happy smile. You are home!

We should have the same good manners toward Nature as we have for each other.
Then, maybe, we will finally stop the destruction we wreak on Her, on our home. HOPEFULLY!
Shanti—Shanti—Shanti—Peace—Peace—Peace

ADVANCED LEVEL 3 LESSON 9

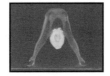

Your mind and body mirror each other. Think about how you "pull yourself together" when you're going to work, out on a date, or in front of a crowd. Then, think about how you "let go" when you're alone. We generally spend our time alternating between these two states of being. In other words, we're generally in a state of over tension, when we're in public, and we're in a collapsed state of being when we are comfortably alone. When we are overly tense, we become uptight, stiff, perhaps hunched up and closed in. On the other hand, when we feel comfortable, in our collapsed state, we are relaxed. Sometimes we can be too relaxed. We slouch, sag, bend forward, and become curved. Both states of being—overly tense and overly collapsed—are unnatural. Both states work against the proper gravity of the body. Both are extremes and, therefore, unhealthy. Regardless of the damage to the body itself, such as a curved or tense spine, both states damage our breathing.

Moving From the Center

If we hold ourselves too stiffly, our lungs do not function properly, and if we slouch not enough air reaches our lungs. When we are healthy, we do not have an upward, pulling tension nor a downward, dragging slackness. We are upright, but relaxed and centered. Our movement is controlled, balanced, even graceful. We can move effortlessly. In complete health, our disposition is also balanced, and we are a pleasure to be around. Outer balance creates inner balance. How many times have you made your body feel good by practicing yoga or by going for a walk? Didn't you find that you also felt better mentally? Haven't you found that when you slouched around at home, your mental attitude also became slouched? Finding the happy medium to these extremes of being means concentrating on being centered. You must learn how to move from your center, breathe from your center, and think from your center. This is called the dan tien, or hara. You can call it anything you wish. It all means that you are centered in the lower abdominal area, about two or three fingers below your navel. This is your energy center. Yoga calls the energy that flows through it prana, the Chinese call it chi, and the Japanese call it ki. It is our life energy center. When it is completely active, it allows a one hundred pound woman to lift a three thousand pound car off a child which has happened. It is the concentrated energy that can be used to chop cement blocks with a bare hand. All martial arts focus on this area, whether it is Karate, Aikido, Kung-Fu, or Tai-Chi Chuan.

Moving from the center is the secret of great power, and good health—both physical and mental. When you stand, you should learn to be rooted, but relaxed. When you move, try to move from your hips, and stop being so dependent on your upper body. Breathe from your center, not from the upper part of your body alone—your lungs and chest area. We generally stand with all our weight on one leg or the other, or with our feet too close together, which is not balanced and makes us very tired. Standing in a balanced position means standing with our feet directly below our hips, our knees slightly relaxed, and our thinking and breathing coming from our center. Try it and notice the difference. You could easily stand like this for hours.

When you go for a walk, try to move from your hip area and from your center. You will find that your walk is more pleasurable and less strenuous. Our body is fairly erect, but as we walk, we tend to lean forward. Have you ever passed a store window and seen the reflection of a hunched over figure and realized it was you? Did you recognize yourself and straighten up right away? Spot check yourself during the day: "How am I standing? How am I moving? How am I breathing?" If you continue to practice this every so often throughout the day, you will soon notice a change in your life. You will become freer, more effortless, flexible, and supple.

When you are centered, you are between heaven and earth. As you move, stand, and think from your center, you unify your body/mind, instead of creating a separation between upper and lower levels. When you live only with the upper or lower part of your body, you're off center. As you find your life's balance, you will also find harmony, and harmony is peace.

In reality, we are always in the center, but we simply don't realize it. Think about where you are sitting at this very moment. There is as much universe to the left of you as there is to the right of you, to the top of you and to the foot of you. Even if you were to move across the room, you'd still be in the center of the universe. Do you see how natural it is to be centered? However, we must have an awareness to feel this centeredness. Stay centered and stay balanced. Change your life and set yourself free.

Continuities

Tell yourself that this is your time to relax. Simply say it to yourself: "This is my time to relax, to really let go, to become empty and open, and to go within." It is more powerful if you say it to yourself, instead of only listening to someone else's words. Learn to give yourself positive thoughts all the time. Get rid of all negativity. Close your eyes and breathe. When you are ready, practice the following continuities in the order listed.

Reclining Continuity

1. Dreaming Dog #1
2. Lie and Stretch #2

3. Leg Raise I and II #3

4. Reverse Bow I and II #4

5. Lying Knees to Floor #35

6. Lying Knee to Head #31

7. Instant Corpse #58

Seated Continuity

1. Sitting Spinal Twist #12

2. Kneeling Reverse Arm Raise #10

3. Camel #29

4. Raised or Leap Frog #83

5. Reverse Frog #21

Standing Continuity

1. Toes, Flat, Chair, Tree #15

2. Standing Waist Roll #51

3. Windmill #52

4. Centered Triangle #74

5. Sun Worship/Sun Salutation #64

6. Standing One Leg Stretch #133

New Postures

Usually, three new postures are introduced in each chapter. In this chapter, however, you will only learn one new posture: Moon Salutation. Like Sun Worship posture, Moon Salutation has multiple positions. There are two primary differences between Sun Worship and Moon Salutation: In Sun Worship, you must hold each position, while in Moon Salutation, your feet remain stationary and your movements are smooth, flowing, and continuous.

158. Moon Salutation (see pp. 248–250).

Stand with your feet spread as wide apart as it is comfortable for you and your toes turned slightly outward. You hands are in front of your abdomen facing upward.

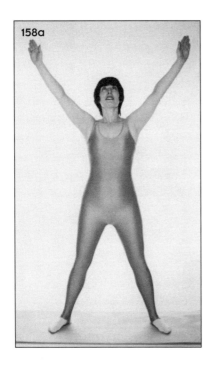

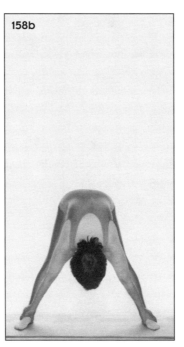

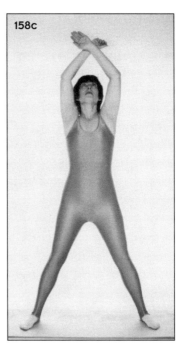

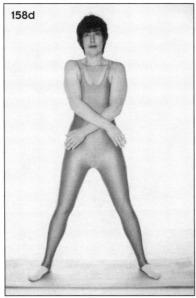

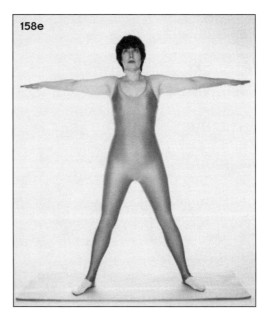

Position One: Inhale and raise your arms up in the air. Your body looks like a big X.

Position Two: Exhale, bend your body forward, and grasp your ankles with your hands.

Position Three: Inhale, raise your body up, and cross your arms over your head.

Position Four: Exhale, lower your arms, and cross them in front of your body.

Position Five: Inhale, raise your arms to the sides at shoulder height.

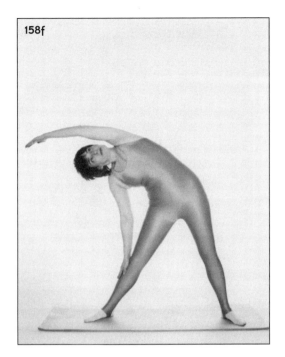

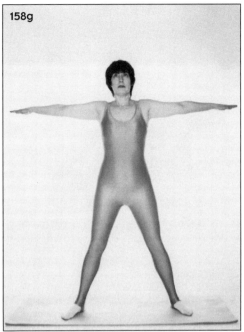

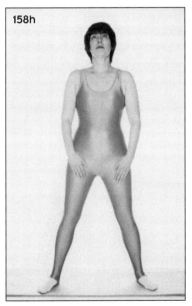

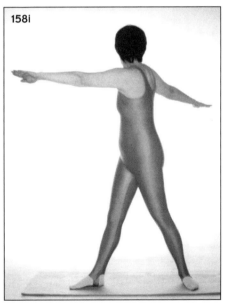

Position Six: Exhale, lean to your right side, and grasp your right ankle with your right hand. Your left arm follows the position of your head, and your elbow is opposite to your ear. Inhale and return to a standing position. Exhale and repeat for the left side of your body.

Position Seven: Inhale and return to a standing position with your arms at shoulder height.

Position Eight: Exhale and lower your arms to the sides.

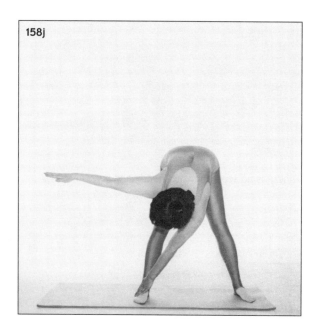

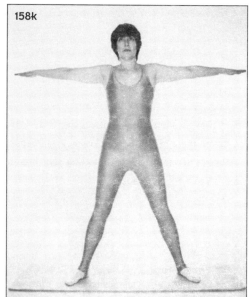

Position Nine: Inhale, raise your arms to shoulder height, and twist your body to the right side. Turn from your waist, and do not twist your knees. Exhale and return to center. Inhale and repeat for the left side of your body. Inhale and return to center, with your arms at shoulder height.

Position Ten: Exhale and twist your body diagonally to the right. Bend down and grasp your right toe with your left hand. Your right arm stays in place. Inhale and lift your body to center. Exhale and repeat for the left side of your body.

Position Eleven: Inhale and lift your body to center with your arms at shoulder height. Exhale and lower your arms to the starting position. Your hands are in front of your abdomen and your palms face upward.

Relaxation/Meditation: Energize and Release

Over the course of this book, you have been through many different types of relaxation/meditation adventures. Some may have been beneficial and rewarding, while others didn't completely fill your needs. You may have found that what works for you one time may not be as effective the next time. However, a practice that didn't work for you once, may prove to be quite helpful the next time. As I mentioned before, we are different each time we practice, and it is important to try different ways of practicing. Regardless of which practice you tried, notice that they all begin with the breath! It is the basis, the groundwork, the door through which we must pass to enter the sublime state. Simply acquainting ourselves with our breath is most important.

Sit as you are for a few moments. Close your eyes and notice your breath. Is it short or is it controlled and relaxed? This is a noticing process so don't try to change your breath, simply witness it, follow it, be aware of it. For the moment, let it follow its own pattern and its own rhythm. This is the spontaneous breath. (Pause.)

Notice that as you become more aware of it, your breath lengthens, slows, and relaxes itself into a more gentle and subtle flow. The longer you follow your breath, the more relaxed, restful, and sleepy you will become. This is one of the initial signs that you are entering meditation. However, if a flood of thoughts enter your mind, then, you have lost your awareness to your breathing. Try to let these thoughts simply pass through, but do not become disturbed by them and do not attach yourself to them. The more you ignore them, the more quickly they will depart.

Begin to concentrate on following your breath, until there is no separation, no breath, and you only breathe! Become it. (Pause.)

Quietly and slowly lie down on the floor. However, instead of lying in a straight, centered, line open yourself up in a large X on the floor. Think of yourself as a large antenna, open and able to pull energy from all corners of the universe. Begin by making sure that your body is relaxed, open to receiving and accepting. Make yourself comfortable now. (Pause.)

As you inhale, think of the word "energize," and as you exhale, think of the word "release." Try it now. (Pause.)

Keep repeating to yourself: energize, release, energize, release. Experience the words taking place within your body with each breath. Feel the energy passing through every fiber of your being, and feel yourself become more and more alive. Then, feel the release take place as your body grows lighter and lighter, no longer weighted down—free! (Pause.)

Imagine that there is an invisible circle drawn around you, connecting your toes and hands. Your torso is the center of the circle. Concentrate more on your inhalation. All the energy that you gather is being stored in your center. Try to feel it now. (Pause.)

Do not try to breathe forcefully. With the proper concentration and awareness, even the most gentle of inhalations will pull the energy inward. (Pause.)

Once you have stored your energy, concentrate more on your exhalation, on the releasing, the letting go, the allowing, and the melting. (Pause.)

Now, think nothing. Only *be!* Be in your *Am*-ness, your *Such*-ness, your *Is*-ness, your *Whole*-ness! You are precious and perfect just as you are at this moment. Experience it, now! (Pause.)

This time, when you bring your body back to aliveness, say your affirmation with more positiveness, more assuredness, and more knowingness than you have ever had before: "My body is relaxed and my mind is peaceful. I am whole and complete just as I am at this moment, and this moment is complete." And, now, stretch as you have never stretched before, as if it were your first time. It is exciting, awesome, and breathtakingly wonderful! When we come to realize that life is a celebration, we will kick up our heels, dance for joy, throw our heads back, and have the deepest belly laugh we have ever had! After your full stretch and your welcomed yawn, try that first laughter and don't ever lose it again!

Any viewing can be sacred, if the viewer is truly seeing.
Stop looking, and SEE!
Shanti—Shanti—Shanti—Peace—Peace—Peace

ADVANCED LEVEL 3 LESSON 10

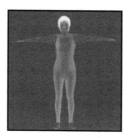

I want to congratulate you for making it this far in your yoga practice. You are to be commended. I applaud you! You should applaud yourself. As I mentioned in the beginning of this book, yoga takes discipline.

What Have You Learned?

You have learned many new postures, many new ways of breathing, and, certainly, much about concentration/meditation. However, what did you really learn? What did you really discover? Hopefully, a little more about truly knowing yourself. You have learned what your body is all about, how to listen to it, move it, how it functions, reacts, and responds, how good it can feel, and does feel, when you treat it properly. You have learned that when you move slowly, gently, and positively, you will be rewarded. You have learned the importance of controlling your breath. You have learned to really let go and relax. You have learned to let the active being in yourself pause, rest, renew, and revive itself. You've turned off your body and mind, and tuned in. After all this, you should know that life doesn't have to be all pain and pressure, fights, flights, and failings. You are learning that it's a floating and flowing, reaping and rewarding, jeweled joy! That lesson has been our goal together, and should continue to be your goal.

 Continuities

Close your eyes and breathe. Relax and begin your postures. Practice the continuities in the order listed.

Seated Continuity

1. Fingers (Raindrops) #100
2. Head Turn and Bend to Side #118
3. Neck Roll #7

4. Turtle #93

5. Shoulder Lift and Roll #8

6. Yoga Triceps Stretch #113

7. Stretch/Open Eyes/Yawn #130

8. Sitting Backward Stretch #36

9. Butterfly and Advanced #19

Standing Continuity

1. Wall Twist #89

2. Side Wall Twist #90

3. Half Moon #91

4. Lateral Stretch #98

5. Moon Stretch #99

6. Sun Worship/Sun Salutation #64

7. Warrior #110

8. Sun Relax #62

9. Headstand #149

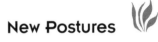

New Postures

Cosmic Breath is a very beautiful, flowing, peaceful posture. In order to obtain the true benefit of the movements, it must be performed at least three times. Most students find that after only three rounds, they feel lighter, more balanced, and more peaceful than with any other posture. Once you have tried it, you will feel changed. As with Moon Salutation, you should not hold each position. The movement should be one continual flow performed very, very slowly and with awareness.

159. Cosmic Breath (see pages 254–256).

Begin by standing in a relaxed, balanced position with your feet under your hips and your arms relaxed by your sides.

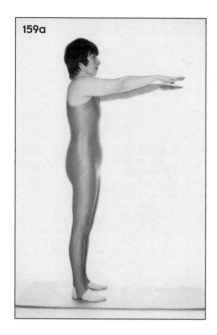

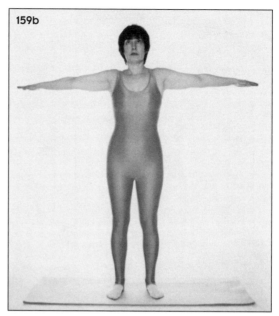

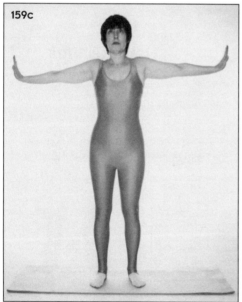

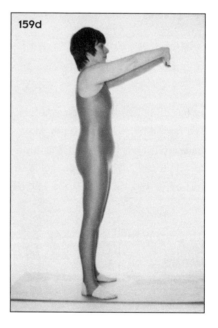

Position One: Inhale and raise your arms in front of you, palms down to shoulder height.

Position Two: Exhale and move your arms to your sides, still at shoulder height and with your palms down.

Position Three: Hold your breath and bend your hands upward at the wrists.

Position Four: Inhale and bring your arms into a circle in front of your face. Your hands are overlapped and their backs are toward your body. Exhale.

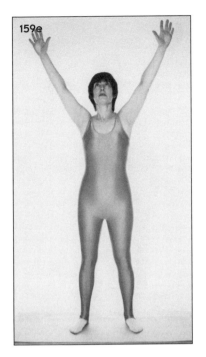

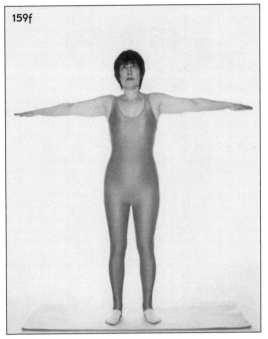

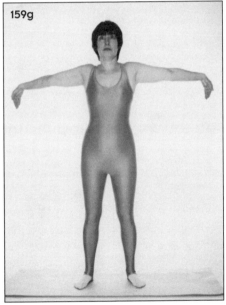

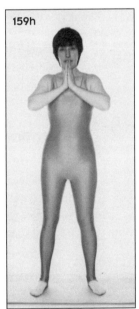

Position Five: Inhale and raise your arms up over your head. Your hands will separate as you raise your arms. Imagine that you are pushing through clouds.

Position Six: Exhale and let your arms float down to shoulder height, palms facing down.

Position Seven: Hold your breath and bend your hands down at the wrists.

Position Eight: Inhale, move your arms forward in a wide circle, and bring your hands under your chin, with your palms together in a prayer position. Exhale.

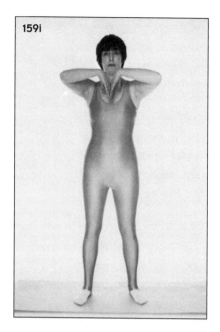

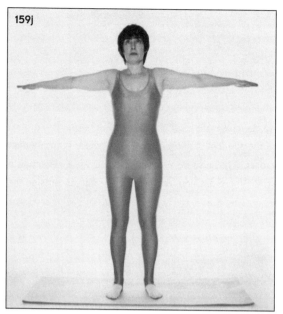

Position Nine: Inhale and lift your elbows. Your hands will separate. Keeping the tips of your fingers touching, roll your hands over your fingers so that the backs are together with your fingers pointing downward. Exhale.

Position Ten: Inhale, open your arms in a wide circle out to the sides at shoulder height, with your palms facing downward. Exhale, let your arms float forward, and cross them in front of your chest. Let your arms relax back to the sides.

Relaxation/Meditation: Raindrop Visualization

We learn that a single raindrop has in its being all the oceans of the world, that we are that single raindrop and that it is us. The so-called difference between us and the raindrop is created by ourselves when we begin to name it. As soon as we name it raindrop, we remove ourselves from it; we create a separation, a division. In so doing, we remove ourselves from the truth.

Let me ask you: If you have an apple pie and take a slice from it is the slice still "apple pie"? It is only your naming it "a slice" that creates the perception of difference? Everything, *everything* is one. There is no division, no separation. The same energy that is the apple, the raindrop, the tree, the locust, the bird is also you. You only need to return to a state of oneness, to open yourself to the beingness of it—the experiencing. Like everything else in life, we sometimes make it more difficult than it is.

Lie down and center yourself in a comfortable position: arms at your sides, legs and back relaxed to the floor, head and neck adjusted correctly. You will begin your journey to beingness.

Take one long, slow inhalation and feel the prana energy flow through every part of your body, filling you with lightness. Slowly exhale and feel the release of any discomfort you may still be holding within you. Let it all go. Let it all flow outward. Inhale again, slowly, with awareness. Feel the air enter your nostrils and flow down into your lungs. Feel it enter your mind—calming it, relaxing it. Exhale slowly and feel your body become more relaxed. Feel your mind become more peaceful—the complete release of all thoughts. You are left with a gentle stillness—quiet and still. (Pause.)

In this stillness, remember once again the single raindrop. Picture it small and perfect, trembling on a leaf. It is poised in the small hollow where the stem connects. It glistens brightly, more iridescent than the most perfect diamond. Look at it.

Move closer to it—closer still. Look inside the raindrop. What do you see? Look closer. Do you see color? Do you see the sunlight shining through it? Where is the sunlight? Is it glowing all through the raindrop? Move closer. What else do you see? Do you see a reflection of yourself looking back at you? Do you see yourself? Where are you, really? Is the real you outside the raindrop looking in or are you inside the raindrop looking out? Are there really two of you or only one? (Pause.)

Look closely. If you wish, you may move inside the raindrop. It's very easy; simply picture yourself on the inside looking out. Are you there? Now, what do you see? What do you feel? Can you see the leaf that you are resting on or can you only see an ocean of green surrounding you? Can you see the sun or do you only see a brilliance of light? Can you feel the heat of the sun as the light flows through you? Can you feel a trembling as the breeze gently ruffles your bed of greenness? Look outward. Can you see another you looking back at you from the outside? Have you become one with the raindrop? Are you the raindrop? Does the raindrop see the ocean of green or do you? Does the raindrop feel the leaf rustle or do you? Does the raindrop feel the heat and light of the sun or do you? Where does the raindrop end and where do you begin? Can you feel any separation, any difference? Have you become the raindrop? Has the raindrop become you? (Pause.)

Feel. Be. Experience. In truth, in oneness there is no division, no separation. We are all that there is, and all that there is, is us. Once we realize this truth, we become overwhelmed with the absolute joy of it, the absolute simplicity of it. It is not difficult at all. It is very simple. It simply is all that is! All we need to do is let go. Let go of all the limitations and restrictions we place on ourselves. We can do it. We already are what we try so hard to be. Stop trying and just be! (Pause.)

Look out again from your raindrop world. Do you see a face looking back at you? Do you see yourself, again out there? It's time to come back to the outside of the raindrop. Take one last look around as you move outward, and bring the feeling of oneness with you. Look back at the raindrop again. The reflection of you is slowly fading. Don't let the experience fade. Keep it with you as you bring your awareness back to your body, to the room around you, to the miracle of this now—this moment. The raindrop will always be with you, whenever you choose to open yourself to the experience of it.

Take a long slow inhalation and fill yourself back to aliveness. Exhale slowly. Inhale and wiggle your arms, your legs, your feet, and your hands. Stretch yourself back to the moment. Feel yourself come alive and allow a wonderful yawn. Remind yourself: "My body is relaxed and my mind is peaceful. I am whole and complete just as I am at this moment." Smile at yourself and at the you in the raindrop.

What we do in this world is our gift to the world.
But HOW we do it is our gift to God!
Shanti—Shanti—Shanti—Peace—Peace—Peace

AFTERWORD

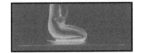

I am always proud and glad for those who complete a course in yoga. It truly is a second chance at life, and everyone should have that chance. Everyone should have a healthy body, a peaceful mind, and spiritual consciousness of truly being. I hope this book has helped you obtain this, for that is my goal in life. You may not have always agreed with what I have told you, which is alright. It simply indicates where you are now. In time, you will understand why I ask you to hug a tree, be totally aware of each moment, and put the ego aside. Until that time comes, keep learning how to stretch to life, how to breathe deeply, how to treat yourself to laughter at least once a day. You'll make it!

Keep reminding yourself that happiness surrounds us in the ten thousand different things. It is not always obvious to the looking, but it is most apparent in the seeing, in awareness to this joyous, wonderful, breathtaking moment of reality that will never come again. The sun greets us warmly in the dawning of the day, but we draw our shades. The bird sings in its morning bath, but we don't stop to truly listen. The colorful flowers, alive with their gentle fragrance, add sweetness to our world, but we don't pause to partake in their gift to us. The breeze that cools us in summer makes the music of dancing leaves in the autumn, but we are deaf to it. The cat purrs upon our lap and the dog licks our hand, but we forget to give thanks for their undying love. The unheralded happiness before us is reason enough to pay attention to each moment just as it is and to be grateful for each moment just as it is! Our lives should be like a flowering, moment to moment, moving from the unseeing sleeping consciousness to a full awakening. Life is counted in, not copping out. It is turning on, not away. It is reaching out and looking in. Life is wholly ours when we see it wholly. It is holy as it is! Surely, life is now and all nows, or it is never.

Why do we dream of a heaven in some future time when it is here now this moment? It is here, if we are aware of it and if we remember to lift our faces to the falling snowflake of winter and to the gentle rain of summer. It is now, if we open ourselves to the melodious sound of raindrops on an upturned bucket, to wind chimes echoing angels' voices, to the hushed hum of waves rolling in. Is it necessary to go down on bended knee in some practiced ritual to be in awe of life? I do not think so. The unpracticed, the ever-new spirit that fills our heart, is far more sincere, more appreciative, and more loving. The happiness of life comes in the spontaneous movement to life grasped wholly. We can throw our heads back and laugh out loud for we will have understood that life is a celebration. You are invited. Come as you are! It's your decision. Will you kick up your heels? Will you curve your lips up in a smile? The decision is always ours. Decide wisely, and begin now, then, continue. Good luck. Stay well and happy. God Bless.

A P P E N D I X

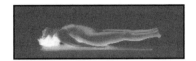

Health Issues, Postures, and Visualizations

Asthma   Corpse pose; Shoulder Stand; Fish; Complete Breath. Visualize lung expansion; renewed strength.

Backache   Corpse pose; Locust; Plow; Knee to Chest. Visualize fresh circulation to nourish back muscles.

Bronchitis   Shoulder Stand (drains out secretions); Fish; Locust.

Cold   Lion; Shoulder Stand.

Constipation Corpse pose; Fish; Twist (loosens spine); Plow; Knee to Chest (reinvigorates liver, spleen, intestines). Visualize increased circulation to tone intestines.

Depression   Shoulder Stand; Plow; Corpse pose. Visualize new energy from increased oxygen; joyous activity.

Diabetes   Corpse pose; Shoulder Stand; Plow (thyroid gland); twist (flexing the spine stimulates nerve impulses to pancreas, massages the pancreas). NOTE: This position aids regulation of diabetes; it is not a cure. Visualize activation of the thyroid gland, which affects the whole metabolism

Emphysema   Complete Breath; Locust; Shoulder Stand. Visualize healing circulation in the lungs.

Eyestrain   Neck and eye exercises (such as the Lion). Visualize absorption of prana energy into the eyes.

Flatulence   Knee to Chest.

Headache	Corpse pose; neck and eye exercises; Shoulder Roll; Neck Roll. Visualize blue summer sky; clear your mind of thought.
Indigestion	Corpse pose; Locust; Shoulder Stand; Plow; Twist; Cobra.
Insomnia	Corpse pose; Locust; Shoulder Stand; Cobra; Infant. Visualize blue sky; clear your mind of thought.
Menstrual	Fish; Cobra; Locust; Pelvic Lift; Triangle.
Neurasthenia	Corpse pose; Shoulder Stand. Visualize energy; giving your bloodstream fresh circulation.
Obesity	Locust; Shoulder Stand; Plow; Cobra; Bow; Sun Salutation.
Piles	Fish; Shoulder Stand; Plow.
Rheumatism	Shoulder Stand; Twist; Knee to Chest. Visualize stiffness in the joints melting away with the dispersal of waste.
Sciatica	Shoulder Stand; Knee to Chest; Plow; Twist.
Sexual debility	Shoulder Stand; Plow; Twist; Complete Breath. Visualize youthful vigor from fresh blood circulation.
Sinus	Neck and eye exercises; Corpse pose; Shoulder Stand.
Skin disease	Sun Salutation. Visualize general physical toning; balancing of irregularity.
Sore throat	Lion. Visualize constricted blood vessels in the throat relaxing, bringing fresh circulation to the sore area.
Varicose veins	Shoulder Stand.
Wrinkles	Shoulder Stand.